A Mom's Guide to the Covid Shot

What Every Mother Needs to Know

Christiane Northrup, M.D.

A Mom's Guide to the Covid Shot: What Every Mother Needs to Know

ISBN 978-1-7364217-6-5

Copyright © 2021 by Christiane Northrup, M.D.

Thrive Publishing

Published by Thrive Publishing

1100 Suite #100 Riverwalk Terrace

Jenks, OK 74037

Thrive Publishing books may be purchased for educational, business or sales promotional use. For more information, please email the Special Markets Department at info@ThriveTimeShow.com. For a good time visit ThriveTimeShow.com

Health and Medical Disclaimer

This book details the author's personal experiences with and opinions about health and wellness. The author is not your healthcare provider.

The author and publisher are providing this book and its contents on an "as is" basis and make no representations or warranties of any kind with respect to this book or its contents. The author and publisher disclaim all such representations and warranties, including for example warranties of merchantability and healthcare for a particular purpose. In addition, the author and publisher do not represent or warrant that the
information accessible via this book is accurate, complete or current.

The statements made about products and services have not been evaluated by the U.S. Food and Drug Administration. They are not intended to diagnose, treat, cure, or prevent any condition or disease. Please consult with your own physician or healthcare specialist regarding the suggestions and recommendations made in this book.

Except as specifically stated in this book, neither the author or publisher, nor any authors, contributors, or other representatives will be liable for damages arising out of or in connection with the use of this book. This is a comprehensive limitation of liability that applies to all damages of any kind, including (without limitation) compensatory; direct, indirect or consequential damages; loss of data, income or profit; loss of ordamage to property and claims of third parties.

You understand that this book is not intended as a substitute for consultation with a licensed healthcare practitioner, such as your physician. Before you begin any healthcare program, or change your lifestyle in any way, you will consult your physician or another licensed healthcare practitioner to ensure that you are in good health and that the examples contained in this book will not harm you.

This book provides content related to physical and/or mental health issues. As such, use of this book implies your acceptance of this disclaimer.

Christiane Northrup, M.D., visionary pioneer in women's health, is a board-certified OB/GYN with more than thirty years of clinical experience, former assistant clinical professor of OB/GYN at the University of Vermont College of Medicine, and three-time *New York Times* bestselling author of *Women's Bodies, Women's Wisdom*, *The Wisdom of Menopause and Goddesses Never Age*. In 2013, *Reader's Digest named Dr. Northrup one of the* "100 Most Trusted People in America." In 2016, she was named one of Oprah Winfrey's Super Soul 100, a group of leaders who are using their voices and talent to awaken humanity. And in 2020 & 2021, she was included in the Watkins Spiritual 100, a list of living people that make a unique and spiritual contribution on a global scale.

Internationally known for her empowering approach, Dr. Northrup embraces medicine that acknowledges the unity of mind, body, emotions, and spirit, and teaches women to create health by tuning into their inner wisdom. After decades spent transforming women's understanding of their sacred bodies and processes, Dr. Northrup now teaches women to thrive at every stage of life.

As a business owner, physician, former surgeon, mother, writer, speaker, and, according to Miriam Ava Ph.D., a "rebel, rock star and authority on what can go right with the female body," Dr. Northrup acknowledges our individual and collective capacity for growth, freedom, joy, and balance.

Dr. Northrup has also hosted eight highly successful public-television specials, and her work has been featured on The Oprah Winfrey Show, the Today Show, NBC Nightly News, The View, Rachael Ray, Good Morning America, 20/20, and The Dr. Oz Show, among many others.

Don't miss Dr. Northrup's cutting-edge information. Join her worldwide community on www.drnorthrup.com, Facebook, Twitter, Telegram, and Instagram.

The current vaccine agenda is based on GERM THEORY <u>only</u> and ignores the contribution of the environment.

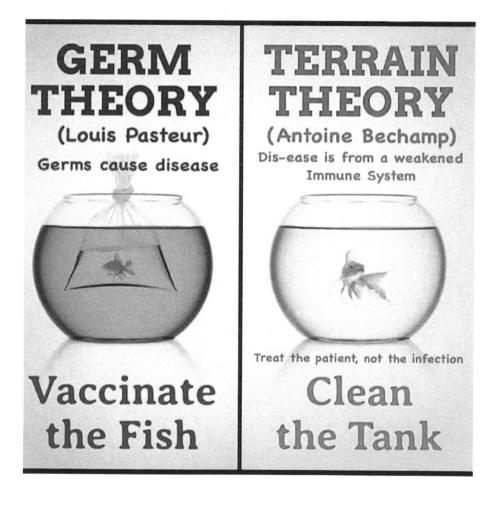

GERM THEORY
(Louis Pasteur)

Germs cause disease

Vaccinate
the Fish

TERRAIN THEORY
(Antoine Bechamp)

Dis-ease is from a weakened
Immune System

Treat the patient, not the infection

Clean
the Tank

Did your doctor tell you to AVOID TUNA when you were pregnant ...

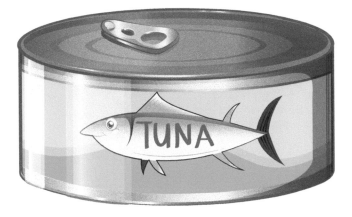

But recommended the flu vaccine?

With ONE SHOT, your child's future and your life could change forever.

It happens...
and there's no turning back.

Thank you for taking empowering steps to become informed and protect your child's health.

To understand the Covid shot, we'll start with a review of the current CDC vaccine schedule for children.

Our children are sicker than ever.

54% now have a chronic disease.*

This needs to stop.

CDC is the Centers for Disease Control and Prevention, a federal agency under Health and Human Services. The CDC decides what vaccines are put on the pediatric vaccine schedule. In some states, kids can't go to school unless they have had all the vaccines on the schedule.

*According to a 2011 survey funded by HHS
https://www.sciencedirect.com/science/article/pii/
S1876285910002500

10

But ...
What Most People Don't Know

"The agencies and people who approve and make vaccines mandatory for the U.S. have received money from vaccine manufacturers.

Think about this and how this corrupts what you are told about vaccines."

- Children's Health Defense, "The FDA, CDC, Media and Politicians Receive Money from Vaccine Makers."

https://childrenshealthdefense.org/vaccine-secrets/video-chapters/the-fda-cdc-media-and-politicians-receive-money-from-vaccine-makers/

CDC Vaccine Schedule
Birth to 18 years of age

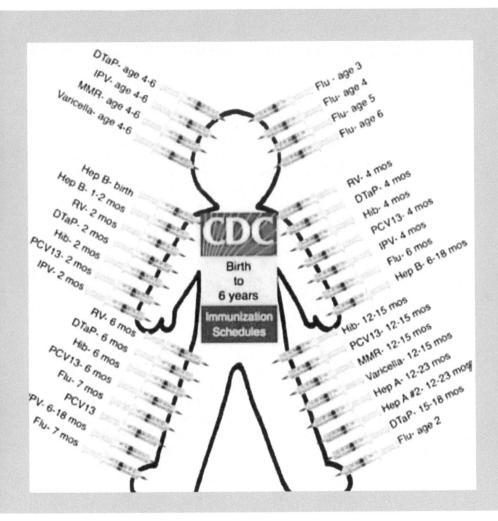

- ## 50 doses of 14 vaccines by age 6

- ## 69 doses of 16 vaccines by age 18

Birth - 15 months

Vaccine	Birth	1 mo	2 mos	4 mos	6 mos	9 mos	12 mos	15 mos
Hepatitis B ⓘ (HepB)	1st dose	←2nd dose→			←3rd dose→			
Rotavirus ⓘ (RV) RV1 (2-dose series); RV5 (3-dose series)			1st dose	2nd dose	See notes			
Diphtheria, tetanus, & acellular pertussis ⓘ (DTaP: <7 yrs)			1st dose	2nd dose	3rd dose			←4th dose→
Haemophilus influenzae type b ⓘ (Hib)			1st dose	2nd dose	See notes		←3rd or 4th dose, See notes→	
Pneumococcal conjugate ⓘ (PCV13)			1st dose	2nd dose	3rd dose		←4th dose→	
Inactivated poliovirus ⓘ (IPV: <18 yrs)			1st dose	2nd dose	←3rd dose→			
Influenza (IIV) ⓘ					Annual vaccination 1 or 2 doses			
or Influenza (LAIV4) ⓘ								
Measles, mumps, rubella ⓘ (MMR)					See notes		←1st dose→	
Varicella ⓘ (VAR)							←1st dose→	
Hepatitis A ⓘ (HepA)					See notes		←2-dose series, See notes→	
Tetanus, diphtheria, & acellular pertussis ⓘ (Tdap: ≥7 yrs)								
Human papillomavirus ⓘ (HPV)								
Meningococcal ⓘ (MenACWY-D ≥9 mos, MenACWY-CRM ≥2 mos, MenACWY-TT ≥2years)			See notes					
Meningococcal B ⓘ (MenB)								
Pneumococcal polysaccharide ⓘ (PPSV23)								

18 months to 18 years

Vaccines	18 mos	19-23 mos	2-3 yrs	4-6 yrs	7-10 yrs	11-12 yrs	13-15 yrs	16 yrs	17-18 yrs
Hepatitis B ⓘ (HepB)	←3rd dose→								
Rotavirus ⓘ (RV) RV1 (2-dose series); RV5 (3-dose series)									
Diphtheria, tetanus, & acellular pertussis ⓘ (DTaP: <7 yrs)	←4th dose→			5th dose					
Haemophilus influenzae type b ⓘ (Hib)									
Pneumococcal conjugate ⓘ (PCV13)									
Inactivated poliovirus ⓘ (IPV: <18 yrs)	←3rd dose→			4th dose					
Influenza (IIV) ⓘ	Annual vaccination 1 or 2 doses				Annual vaccination 1 dose only				
or Influenza (LAIV4) ⓘ			Annual vaccination 1 or 2 doses		or Annual vaccination 1 dose only				
Measles, mumps, rubella ⓘ (MMR)				2nd dose					
Varicella ⓘ (VAR)				2nd dose					
Hepatitis A ⓘ (HepA)	← 2-dose series, See notes→								
Tetanus, diphtheria, & acellular pertussis ⓘ (Tdap: ≥7 yrs)						Tdap			
Human papillomavirus ⓘ (HPV)					★	See notes			
Meningococcal ⓘ (MenACWY-D ≥9 mos, MenACWY-CRM ≥2 mos, MenACWY-TT ≥2years)	See notes					1st dose		2nd dose	
Meningococcal B ⓘ (MenB)							See notes		
Pneumococcal polysaccharide ⓘ (PPSV23)				See notes					

What's in a vaccine?

Vaccines contain toxic and dangerous ingredients. Small doses can cause harm.

Aluminum
known neurotoxin

Aborted fetal tissue
cancer concern

Mercury
known neurotoxin

"New CDC Research Debunks Agency's Assertion That Mercury in Vaccines Is Safe" - Children's Health Defense

https://childrenshealthdefense.org/news/new-cdc-research-debunks-agenoys-assertion-that-mercury-in-vaccines-is-safe/

Vaccine

VIRUS

Ingredients in Hep B (Hepatitus B)

Given at Birth

formaldehyde, potassium **aluminum** sulfate, amorphous **aluminum** hydroxyphosphate sulfate, yeast protein

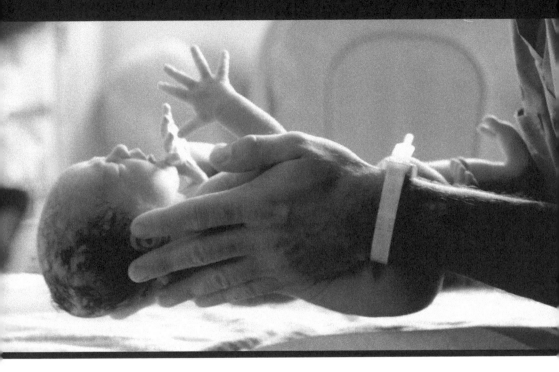

Formaldehyde
Formaldehyde is highly toxic and is an eye, skin, and respiratory tract irritant.

Aluminum
Aluminum is well known as a neurotoxin and may be associated with Alzheimer's disease.

Hep B vaccine contains unsafe levels of aluminum.

https://www.rescuepost.com/files/exley-commentary.pdf
https://www.cdc.gov/vaccines/pubs/pinkbook/downloads/appendices/B/excipient-table-2.pdf

Ingredients in MMR (MMR-II)

Measles, Mumps, Rubella

vitamins, amino acids, fetal bovine serum, sucrose, glutamate, recombinant human albumin, neomycin, sorbitol, hydrolyzed gelatin, sodium phosphate, sodium chloride, **WI-38 human diploid lung fibroblasts**

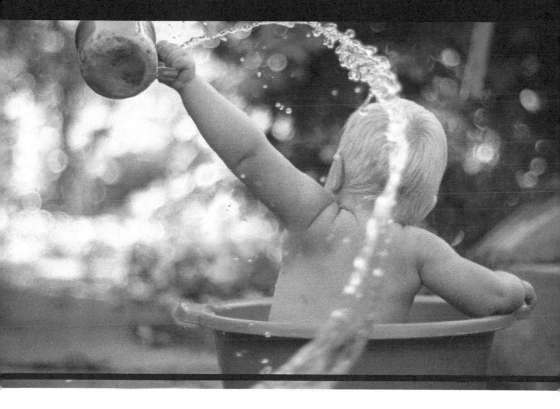

 ## WI-38 human diploid lung fibroblasts

Aborted fetal tissue
The WI-38 human diploid cell line was derived by Leonard Hayflick from normal embryonic **(3 months gestation)** lung tissue.

https://www.cdc.gov/vaccines/pubs/pinkbook/downloads/appendices/B/excipient-table-2.pdf

Things That Can Go Wrong

ADVERSE REACTIONS - MMRII

The following adverse reactions include those identified during clinical trials or reported during post-approval use of M-M-R II vaccine or its individual components.

Body as a Whole
Panniculitis; atypical measles; fever; syncope; headache; dizziness; malaise; irritability.

Cardiovascular System
Vasculitis. Digestive System Pancreatitis; diarrhea; vomiting; parotitis; nausea.

Hematologic and Lymphatic Systems
Thrombocytopenia; purpura; regional lymphadenopathy; leukocytosis.

Immune System
Anaphylaxis, anaphylactoid reactions, angioedema (including peripheral or facial edema) and bronchial spasm.

Musculoskeletal System
Arthritis; arthralgia; myalgia.

More Things That Can Go Wrong

The following adverse reactions include those identified during clinical trials or reported during post-approval use of M-M-R II vaccine or its individual components.

Nervous System Encephalitis
Encephalopathy; measles inclusion body encephalitis (MIBE) subacute sclerosing panencephalitis (SSPE); Guillain-Barré Syndrome (GBS); acute disseminated encephalomyelitis (ADEM); transverse myelitis; febrile convulsions; afebrile convulsions or seizures; ataxia; polyneuritis; polyneuropathy; ocular palsies; paresthesia.

Respiratory System
Pneumonia; pneumonitis; sore throat; cough; rhinitis.

Skin
Stevens-Johnson syndrome; acute hemorrhagic edema of infancy; Henoch-Schönlein purpura; erythema multiforme; urticaria; rash; measles-like rash; pruritus; injection site reactions (pain, erythema, swelling and vesiculation).

Special Senses Ear Nerve deafness; otitis media.

Special Senses Eye Retinitis; optic neuritis; papillitis; conjunctivitis.

Urogenital System Epididymitis; orchitis.

https://www.fda.gov/media/75191/download

19

MMR and the CDC Whistleblower

On August 27th, 2014, a senior scientist at the Centers for Disease Control and Prevention (CDC), Dr. William Thompson released this statement,

"I regret that my coauthors and I omitted statistically significant information in our 2004 article published in the journal *Pediatrics*.

The omitted data suggested that African American males who received the MMR vaccine before age 36 months were at increased risk for autism.

Decisions were made regarding which findings to report after the data were collected, and I believe that the final study protocol was not followed."

Press Release from Morgan Verkamp, LLC.

 Medical Racism: The New Apartheid
Exposing the Truth Behind Systemic Racism in Medicine
https://medicalracism.childrenshealthdefense.org/

https://legislature.vermont.gov/Documents/2016/WorkGroups/House%20Health%20Care/Bills/H.98/
Witness%20Testimony/H.98~Jennifer%20Stella~William%20Thompson%20Statement~5-6-2015.pdf

Black boys who received the MMR vaccine *prior to three years old* were **3.36 times** more likely to receive an autism diagnosis than those who received the vaccine after 3 years of age.

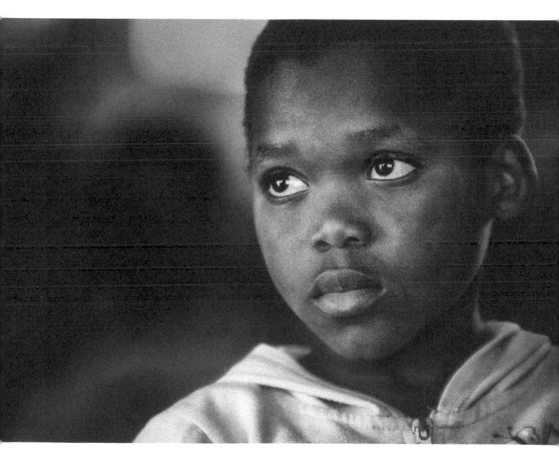

The HPV Vaccine On Trial
Seeking Justice For A Generation Betrayed

A Must-Read Book for All Parents

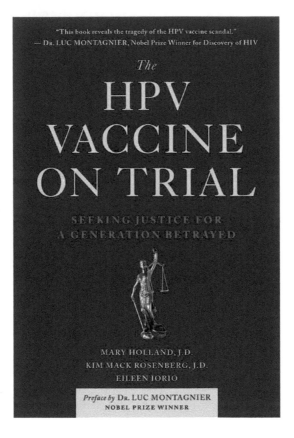

"No parent should make the decision to vaccinate their child until they have read and understood this book."

—Jonathan Irwin

Founder, The Jack & Jill Foundation Ireland,
Former racetrack executive,
Parent of a child who reacted adversely
to the HPV vaccine.

"I have voiced concerns about this vaccine from the time it first got fast tracked through the system and even spoke out about it on an Oprah appearance years ago. Finally the whole story is revealed in this book. It is high time."

—Christiane Northrup, MD

Author of *Women's Bodies, Women's Wisdom*

https://www.simonandschuster.com/books/The-HPV-Vaccine-On-Trial/Mary-Holland/9781510710801

If you or your child has a vaccine injury,

you get left with all the bills!

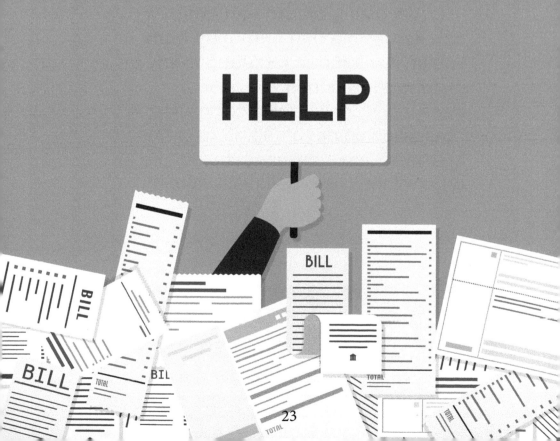

Why Phamaceutical Companies have NO REASON to make their Products Safe

"In 1986, Congress passed the National Childhood Vaccine Injury Act (NCVIA), **giving pharmaceutical companies blanket immunity from liability for injuries resulting from childhood vaccines.**The liability protections converted vaccines from a "neglected corner of the drugs business" into a major economic driver of the pharmaceutical industry."

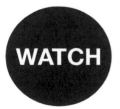

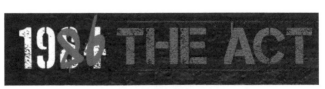

https://7thchakrafilms.com/

U.S. Autism Rates Up in New CDC Report

1 in 54

2000 **1 in 150**

U.S. Centers for Disease Control and Prevention

https://www.cdc.gov/ncbddd/autism/data.html

25

Vaccinated vs. Unvaccinated
Who's Healthier?

"Ten-Year Study: Unvaccinated Children Far Healthier Than Their Vaccinated Peers."

- No ADHD in the unvaccinated

- Unvaccinated had 25 times fewer pediatric visits

- Vaccinated children up to six times more likely to suffer from anemia, allergies, sinusitis, and asthma

"DTP Vaccine Increases Mortality in Young Infants 5 to 10-fold compared to unvaccinated infants."

- All currently available evidence suggests that DTP vaccine may kill more children from other causes than it saves from diphtheria, tetanus or pertussis.

https://childrenshealthdefense.org/news/dtp-vaccine-increases-mortality-in-young-infants-5-to-10-fold-compared-to-unvaccinated-infants/

https://nationalvanguard.org/2020/12/ten-year-study-unvaccinated-children-far-healthier-than-their-vaccinated-peers/

5 Must-Know Tips

1. Read the package insert including all fine print.

2. Read the Vaccine Information Statement (VIS).

3. Know the side effects and the time period in which each side effect must take place to show that the vaccine caused the reaction.
See the Vaccine Injury Table at Health Resources and Services Administration (HRSA).

4. Keep a written record of the vaccine manufacturer's name and lot number.

5. Know how to identify and report a vaccine reaction.

Getting a flu shot increases your risk of getting Coronavirus by

36%.

"Pentagon Study: Flu Shot Raises Risk of Coronavirus by 36% (and Other Supporting Studies)",

Robert F. Kennedy, Jr., April 16, 2020.

What's in the Covid Shots?

ING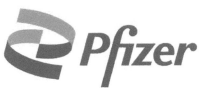NTS

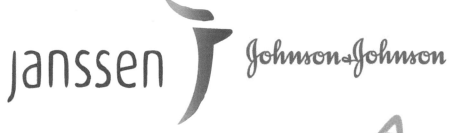

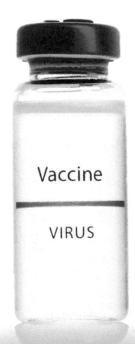

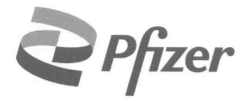

mRNA, lipids ((4-hydroxybutyl)azanediyl)bis(hexane-6,1-diyl)bis(2-hexyldecanoate), 2 [(polyethylene glycol)-2000]-N,N-ditetradecylacetamide, 1,2-Distearoyl-sn-glycero-3-phosphocholine, and cholesterol), potassium chloride, monobasic potassium phosphate, sodium chloride, dibasic sodium phosphate dihydrate, and sucrose.

moderna

messenger ribonucleic acid (mRNA), lipids (SM-102, polyethylene glycol [PEG] 2000 dimyristoyl glycerol [DMG], cholesterol, and 1,2-distearoyl-sn-glycero-3-phosphocholine [DSPC]), tromethamine, tromethamine hydrochloride, acetic acid, sodium acetate trihydrate, and sucrose.

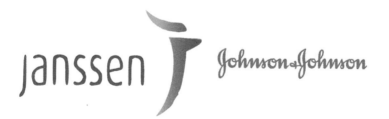

recombinant, replication-incompetent adenovirus type 26 expressing the SARS-CoV-2 spike protein, citric acid monohydrate, trisodium citrate dihydrate, ethanol, 2-hydroxypropyl-β-cyclodextrin (HBCD), polysorbate-80, sodium chloride.

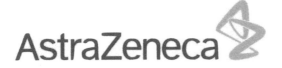

Recombinant, replication-deficient chimpanzee adenovirus vector encoding the SARS-CoV-2 Spike (S) glycoprotein (GP).

The vaccine is manufactured using material originally sourced from a human embryo (Human Embryonic Kidney cells: HEK293).

COVID-19 Vaccine AstraZeneca contains the excipients histidine, histidine hydrochloride monohydrate, sodium chloride, magnesium chloride hexahydrate, disodium edetate (EDTA), sucrose, ethanol absolute, polysorbate 80 and water for injections.

Brand NEW Technologies

Humans are the Test Subjects

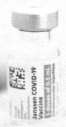

mRNA

"This [mRNA] is the critical information that determines what the cell will do.

So we think about it as an

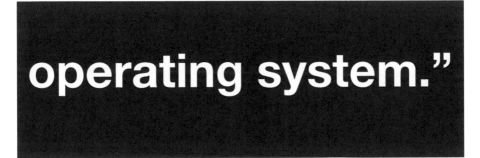

operating system."

Dr. Tal Zaks
Chief Medical Officer at Moderna Inc.
2017 TED talk

https://www.youtube.com/watch?v=FU-cqTNQhMM
https://vaccineimpact.com/2021/the-new-mrna-covid-vaccines-inject-an-operating-system-into-your-body-not-a-conspiracy-theory-moderna-admits-it/

mRNA instructs cells to create the Spike Protein.

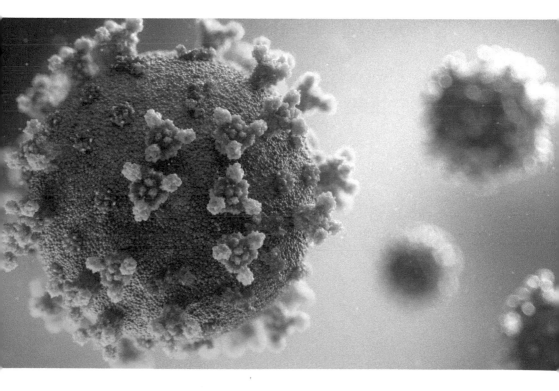

GGGAAATAAGAGAGAAAGAAGAGTAAGAAGAAATATAAGACCCCGGCGCCGCCACCATGTTCGTGTTCCTGGTGC
GCCCCTGGTGAGCAGCCAGTGCGTGAACCTGACCACCCGGACCCAGCTGCCACCAGCCTACACCAACAGCTTCACC
GCGTCTACTACCCCGACAAGGTGTTCCGGAGCAGCGTCCTGCACAGCACCCAGGACCTGTTCCTGCCCTTCTTCAG
GTGACCTGGTTCCACGCCATCCACGTGAGCGGCACCAACGGCACCAAGCGGTTCGACAACCCCGTGCTGCCCTTCA
CGGCGTGTACTTCGCCAGCACCGAGAAGAGCAACATCATCCGGGGCTGGATCTTCGGCACCACCCTGGACAGCAAG

This is
synthetic mRNA

It really is like
software code

TGTGCGAGTTCCAGTTCTGCAACGACCCCTT
TTCCGGGTGTACAGCAGCGCCAACAACTGCA
GGGCAACTTCAAGAACCTGCGGGAGTTCGTG
TCAACCTGGTGCGGGATCTGCCCCAGGGCTT
CGGTTCCAGACCCTGCTGGCCCTGCACCGGA
TGCTTACTACGTGGGCTACCTGCAGCCCCGG
ACTGCGCCCTGGACCCTCTGAGCGAGACCAA
AACTTCCGGGTGCAGCCCACCGAGAGCATCG
CGCCACCCGGTTCGCCAGCGTGTACGCCTGG
ACAGCGCCAGCTTCAGCACCTTCAAGTGCTA
GCCGACAGCTTCGTGATCCGTGGCGACGAGC
CAAGCTGCCCGACGACTTCACCGGCTGCGTC
ACTACCTGTACCGGCTGTTCCGGAAGAGCAA
TCCACCCCTTGCAACGGCGTGGAGGGCTTCA
GGGCTACCAGCCCTACCGGGTGGTGGTGCTC
GCACCAACCTGGTGAAGAACAAGTGCGTGAA
AAGAAATTCCTGCCCCTTTCAGCAGTTCGGCC
GATCCTGGACATCACCCCTTGCAGCTTCGGC
TGCTGTACCAGGACGTGAACTGCACCGAGGT
AGCACCGGCAGCAACGTGTTCCAGACCCGGC
CATCCCCATCGGCGCCGGCATCTGTGCCAGC
AGAGCATCATCGCCTACACCATGAGCCTGGC
AACTTCACCATCAGCGTGACCACCGAGATTC
CGGCGACAGCACCGAGTGCAGCAACCTGCTC
TCGCCGTGGGAGCAGGACAAGAACACCCAGGA
TTCGGCGGCTTCAACTTCAGCCAGATCCTGC
CAACAAGGTGACCCTAGCCGACGCCGGCTTC
TCTGCGCCCAGAAGTTCAACGGCCTGACCGT
CTGTTAGCCGGAACCATCACCAGCGGCTGGA
CTACCGGTTCAACGGCATCGGCGTGACCCAC
CCATCGGCAAGATCCAGGACAGCCTGAGCAC
CAGGCCCTGAACACCCTGGTGAAGCAGCTGA
GCTGGACCCTCCCGAGGCCGAGGTGCAGATC
AGCAGCTGATCCGGGCCGCCGAGATTCGGGC

GCCAACCTGGCCGCCACCAAGATGAGCGAGTGCGTGCTGGGCCAGAGCAAGCGGGTGGACTTCTGCGGCAAGGGC
CCTGATGAGCTTTCCCCAGAGCGCACCCCACGGAGTGGTGTTCCTGCACGTGACCTACGTGCCCGCCCAGGAGAA
TCACCACCGCCCCAGCCATCTGCCACGACGGCAAGGCCCACTTTCCCCGGGAGGGCGTGTTCGTGAGCAACGGCA
TGGTTCGTGACCCAGCGGAACTTCTACGAGCCCCAGATCATCACCACCGACAACACCTTCGTGAGCGGCAACTGC
GGTGATCGGCATCGTGAACAACACCGTGTACGATCCCCTGCAGCCCGAGCTGGACAGCTTCAAGGAGGAGCTGGA
ACTTCAAGAATCACACCAGCCCCGACGTGGACCTGGGCGACATCAGCGGCATCAACGCCAGCGTGGTGAACATCC
GAGATCGATCGGCTGAACGAGGTGGCCAAGAACCTGAACGAGAGCCTGATCGACCTGCAGGAGCTGGGCAAGTAC
GTACATCAAGTGGCCCTGGTACATCTGGCTGGGCTTCATCGCCGGCCTGATCGCCATCGTGATGGTGACCATCAT

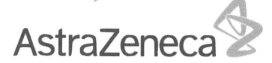

AstraZeneca uses a chimpanzee adenovirus. Janssen is based on a human adenovirus.

The AD26.COV2.S vaccine utilizes adenovirus technology to expose human immune systems to SARS-CoV-2 virus antigens. This is achieved by **cloning a copy of DNA** that encodes the SARS-CoV-2 spike protein into a loop of DNA called a plasmid, which is then housed within a modified adenovirus.

Once introduced into the body, the modified adenovirus binds and enters human cells. At this point, the body of the virus essentially disintegrates, allowing the **genetic material within to travel into the nucleus of human cells.** Once there, native enzymes that transcribe DNA into mRNA take over and start to turn out strips of mRNA that code for the spike proteins. These mRNA strips — called *transcripts* — are then translated into the spike protein. Finally, the spike proteins are then packed and sent to the outer cell membrane where they can be accessed by the host immune system.

https://coronavirus.medium.com/decoding-johnson-johnsons-covid-19-vaccine-ingredients-42a65aa814eb

"We are actually hacking the software of life."

Dr. Tal Zaks
Chief Medical Officer at Moderna Inc.
2017 TED talk

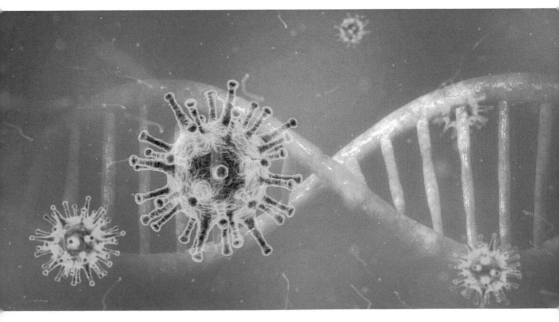

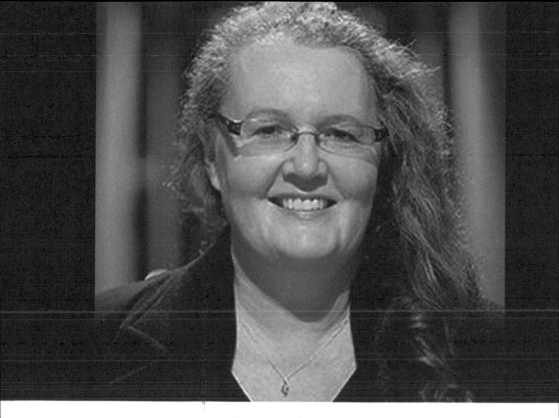

Dolores Cahill Ph.D.
Molecular Biologist/Immunologist

"

When you inject it, this mRNA, why it's so deadly, is that it now goes into your genes and starts expressing.

And it **starts stimulating the immune response from inside your body, and you can't get rid of it** because of the source of the viral protein.

You now have become like a

genetically modified organism.

Spike Protein Disrupts the Blood-Brain Barrier

The SPIKE PROTEIN in itself creates disease

● **American Heart Association**

"SARS-CoV-2 Spike Protein Impairs Endothelial Function via Downregulation of ACE 2."

● **The Salk Institute**

"The Novel Coronavirus' Spike Protein Plays Additional Key Role in Illness."

The AHA study "rescue treatment" used N-acetyl-L-cysteine (NAC), a reactive oxygen species inhibitor.

https://www.ahajournals.org/doi/10.1161/CIRCRESAHA.121.318902
https://www.salk.edu/news-release/the-novel-coronavirus-spike-protein-plays-additional-key-role-in-illness/

How many SPIKE PROTEINS are in a shot?

50 Billion

Janssen and AstraZeneca

Other Ingredients of Concern
Ingredients are never One-Size Fits-All

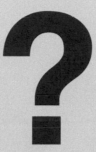

Are you OK with having polyethylene glycol injected into your body?

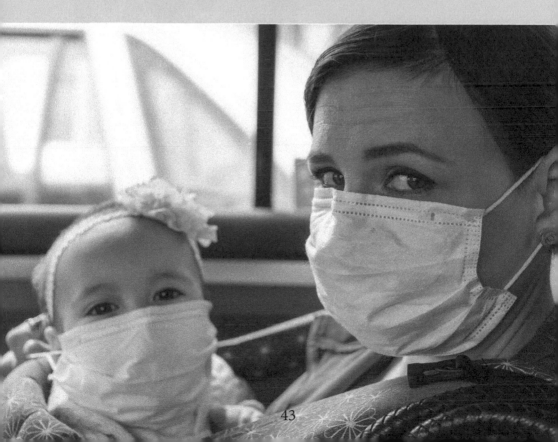

PEG   Polyethylene glycol

The Lipid Nanoparticles (LNPs) that encapsulate mRNA contain PEG

Danger
of Anaphylaxis

70%

2016

"Seventy percent of people make antibodies to PEG and most do not know it, creating a concerning situation where many could have allergic, potentially deadly, reactions to a PEG-containing vaccine."

\- Dr. Michael Yeadon
and Dr. Wolfgang Wodarg

1970   **0.2%**

https://dryburgh.com/wp-content/uploads/2020/12/
Wodarg_Yeadon_EMA_Petition_Pfizer_Trial_FINAL_01DEC2020_signed_with_Exhibits_geschwarzt.pdf

Thousands of Products contain PEG

- Soap
- Sunblock
- Detergent
- Processed Foods
- Toothpaste

- Shampoo
- Cosmetics
- Laxatives
- Colonoscopy Prep
- e-cigarettes

- FDA approved medications (1,155)

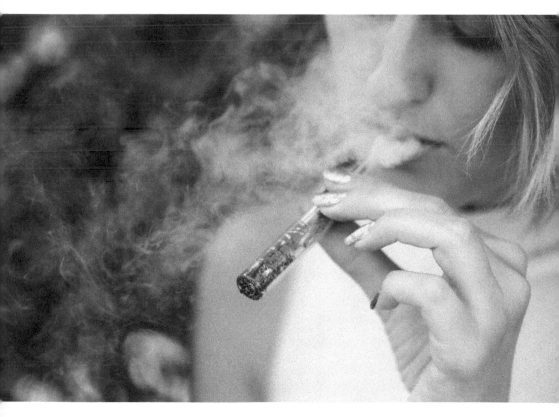

Polysorbate 80

Johnson & Johnson Janssen Vaccine

Allows uptake of drugs across the normally protective blood-brain barrier.

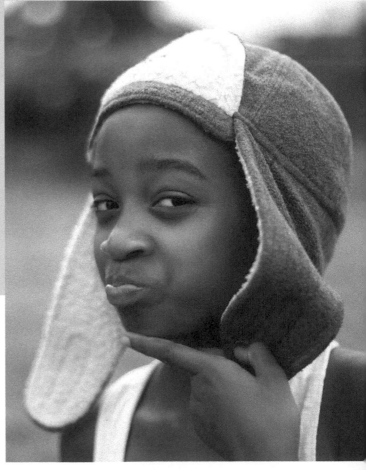

https://www.sciencedirect.com/science/article/abs/pii/0378517389902664

F t l Cell Lin s

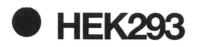

HEK293 Moderna, Pfizer, AstraZeneca

"Scientists harvested this cell line from the kidney of a female Dutch fetus legally aborted in 1973 and then immortalized the cells by rendering them cancerous."

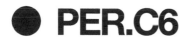

PER.C6 Johnson & Johnson Janssen Vaccine

"Researchers harvested these cell lines from the eyeball of an 18-week-old human fetus aborted in 1985, and then rendered them Immortal by making them cancerous."

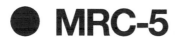

MRC-5 AstraZeneca

"The cell line was derived from the human lung tissue of a 14-week-old male fetus aborted from a 27-year-old woman."

https://childrenshealthdefense.org/defender/fda-cancer-cells-in-vaccines/
https://www.tga.gov.au/sites/default/files/cmi-approved-covid19-vaccine-az.pdf
https://micro.magnet.fsu.edu/primer/techniques/fluorescence/gallery/cells/mrc5/mrc5cells.html
https://web.archive.org/web/20170516050447/https://www.fda.gov/ohrms/dockets/ac/01/transcripts/3750t1_01.pdf

The Cancer Concern

"Is it relevant to safety that a cell forms a tumor after a year, a year-and-a-half?"

Dr. Keith Peden

Office of Vaccines at CBER, Division of Viral Products

According to FDA's **"The Pink Sheet"** dated Nov. 29, 1999, for two decades the agency has been acutely aware of the inherent risks of using immortalized cell lines for vaccine development. The FDA CBER Director, Dr. Peter Patriarca, M.D., explained that continuous cell lines are used for their ability to self-propagate, making them an ideal substrate on which to grow viruses, **"the worst thing we are concerned about is malignancy, because some of these continuous cells have the potential for growing tumors in laboratory animals."**

https://childrenshealthdefense.org/defender/fda-cancer-cells-in-vaccines/
https://www.crisismagazine.com/wp-content/uploads/2021/04/Van-Ep-talk-on-Origin-of-HEK293-see-p-77ff.pdf

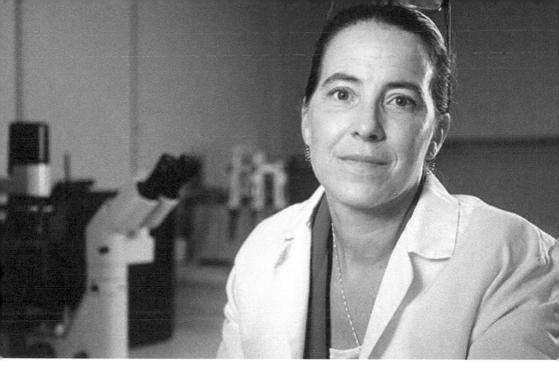

Theresa A. Deisher, Ph.D.

President, Sound Choice Pharmaceutical Institute , CEO and Managing Member, AVM Biotechnology. Expert in the field of adult stem cell therapies and regenerative medicine.

Human DNA in Vaccines

"No final drug is ever completely 'pure' and you will find **contaminating DNA and cellular debris** from the production cell **in your final product.**"

https://bioethicsarchive.georgetown.edu/pcbe/transcripts/sept08/deisher_statement.pdf

The full health
implications of the use
of fetal cell lines in
vaccines is

unknown.

mNeonGreen and Luciferase

- Bioluminescent qualities

- Typically used for medical imaging purposes

- Has never been used in a vaccine before.

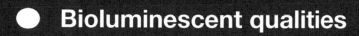
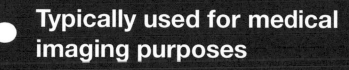

"Pfizer/BioNTech is also inserting an ingredient derived from a marine invertebrate, **mNeonGreen**, into its vaccine. The ingredient has bioluminescent qualities, making it attractive for medical imaging purposes, but

it is unclear why an injected vaccine would need to have that quality.

mNeonGreen has unknown antigenicity."

Dr. Michael Yeadon, Dr. Wolfgang Wodarg
in Petition to European Medicines Agency

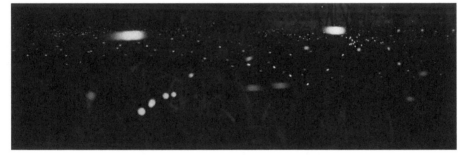

Lampyridae - Fireflies

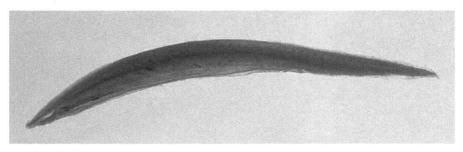

Branchiostoma lanceolatum - Marine Invertebrate

SM-102

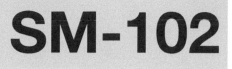
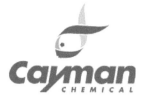

PRODUCT INFORMATION

Description

SM-102 is an ionizable amino lipid that has been used in combination with other lipids in the formation of lipid nanoparticles.[1] Administration of luciferase mRNA in SM-102-containing lipid nanoparticles induces hepatic luciferase expression in mice. Formulations containing SM-102 have been used in the development of lipid nanoparticles for delivery of mRNA-based vaccines.

> **WARNING**
> **THIS PRODUCT IS FOR RESEARCH ONLY - NOT FOR HUMAN OR VETERINARY DIAGNOSTIC OR THERAPEUTIC USE.**

https://www.caymanchem.com/pdfs/33474.pdf

Cayman Chem Company Statement
SM-102 for Research Use Only (RUO)
5/19/21

> **RUO–grade products, such as Cayman's** SM–102 (Item # 33474)**, are intended only for in vitro or animal (exploratory or preclinical) use.**

https://www.caymanchem.com/news/sm-102-statement

IT'S MAGNETIC!!!

Is this why?

New Discovery:
"Genetically engineered
'Magneto' protein remotely
controls brain and behaviour."

https://www.theguardian.com/science/neurophilosophy/2016/mar/
24/magneto-remotely-controls-brain-and-behaviour

https://ugetube.com/watch/magnet-challenge-tested-on-random-people-laguna-beach-california-
highwire-covid-19-coronavirus-masks_Kh5vac6fo7FzZN1.html

Magnetized Iron Nanoparticles

Study

"Superparamagnetic nanoparticle delivery of DNA vaccine"

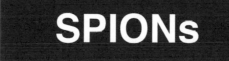

superparamagnetic iron oxide nanoparticles

"The efficiency of delivery of DNA vaccines is often relatively low compared to protein vaccines. The use of superparamagnetic iron oxide nanoparticles (SPIONs) **to deliver genes via magnetofection** shows promise in improving the efficiency of gene delivery both in vitro and in vivo."

Hydrogel

PEG derivatives are largely employed in the formation of hydrogels.

"These nanoparticles can **replicate inside the body**-
theoretically they could be transmissible in some way.
Bacteria/bacteriophages can make the materials needed
to help the nanoparticles reproduce - particularly "hydrogel".

Hydrogel can bind to the nervous system and become a
hybrid organic tissue/synthetic tissue"

Dr. Carrie Madej
Osteopathic Internal Medicine Physician

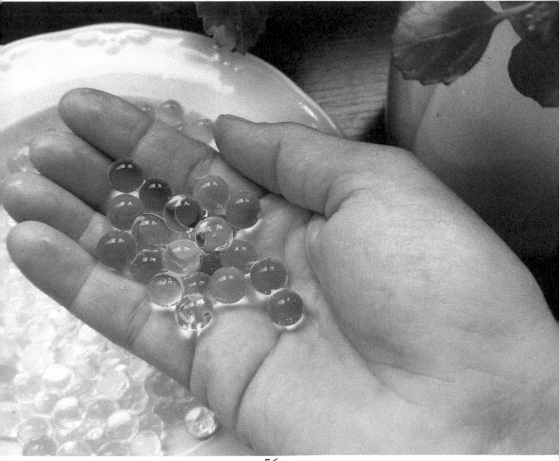

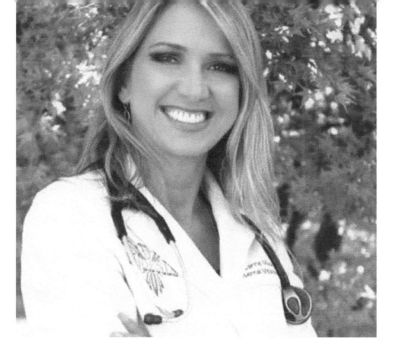

Dr. Carrie Madej
Osteopathic Internal Medicine Physician

" You can't receive a patent for anything natural or from nature. But you can patent anything that has been created, modified or engineered.

U.S. Supreme Court 2013 Ruling on Synthetic Genes

So when this gets into the genome, if it's permanent, guess what?

You, as a human, can be patented and owned.

https://www.supremecourt.gov/opinions/12pdf/12-398_1b7d.pdf
https://ourgreaterdestiny.org/2021/01/gene-altering-mrna-covid-vax-warning-dr-carrie-madej/

New Ways To Deliver Drugs/Vaccines

From hydrogel nanoparticles for nasal delivery to micro theragrippers

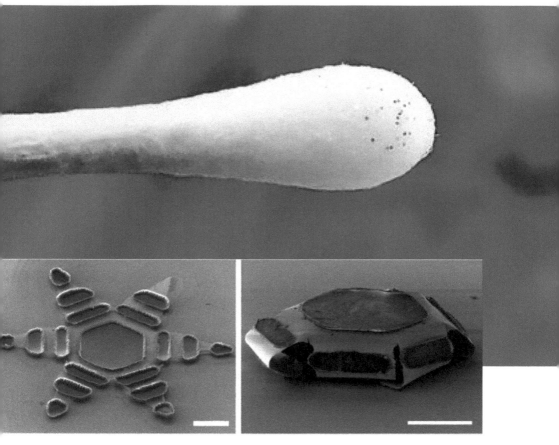

Micro Theragrippers - Johns Hopkins University
Photo: Johns Hopkins University

Studies

"Hydrogel nanoparticles and nanocomposites for nasal drug/vaccine delivery"

"Gastrointestinal-resident, shape-changing microdevices extend drug release in vivo"

 Did you ever wonder why people were told to wear a mask to stop viral particles but a PCR test swab had to be inserted far into their nasal cavity to get a sample?

https://advances.sciencemag.org/content/6/44/eabb4133.full
https://link.springer.com/article/10.1007%2Fs12272-016-0782-0

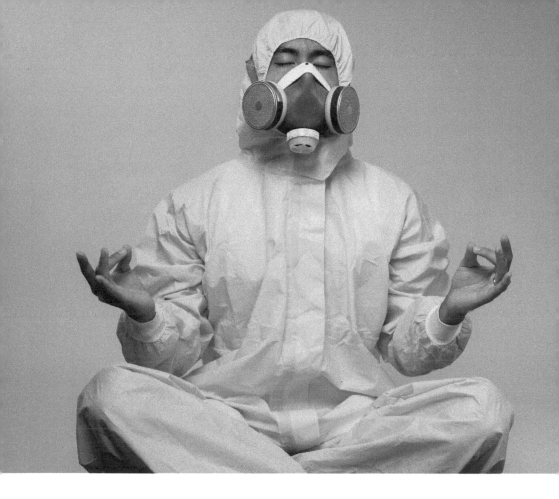

Ready
for More
Truth?

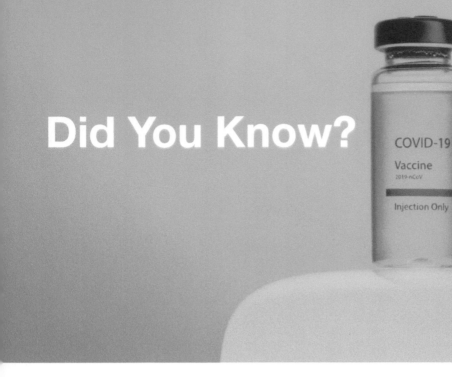

Did You Know?

The Covid Vaccines

are not Vaccines at all

Legal Definition of a Vaccine

Under CDC and FDA standards a vaccine must meet **both** of these criteria:

 It must stimulate an immunity within the person receiving it.

 It must disrupt transmission.

Dr. David E. Martin
"This is Not A Vaccine! It is a Medical Device."

https://leohohmann.com/2021/03/12/heres-why-mrna-injections-do-not-meet-the-legal-definition-of-vaccine/

The COVID-19 vaccine is an *experimental* medical protocol authorized under the Emergency Authorization Act

They are NOT FDA-Approved.

Average number of years to produce a vaccine

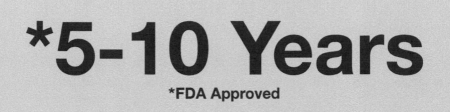

*5-10 Years

*FDA Approved

Length of time to produce the COVID-19 Vaccine

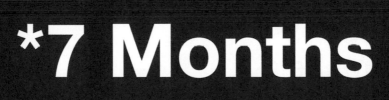

*7 Months

*Emergency Use Authorization Only

5/15/20 - Operation Warp Speed announced
12/11/20 - FDA gives Pfizer EUA authorization

https://thehill.com/opinion/white-house/544175-getting-the-facts-right-on-operation-warp-speed

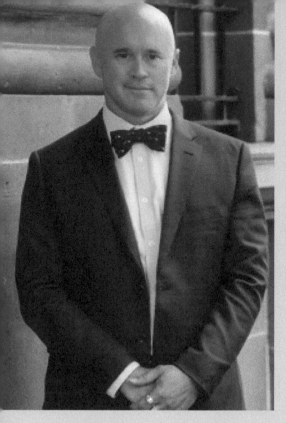

"This is **a mechanical device** in the form of a very small packet of technology that is being inserted into the human system to activate the cell to become a pathogen-manufacturing site."

"A vaccine is supposed to trigger immunity.

It's not supposed to trigger you to make a toxin."

Dr. David E. Martin

Corporate Advisor I Entrepreneur I Financier I Storyteller I Professor I Inventor

"Clinicians have been telling me that **more than half** of the new COVID cases that they're treating are **people who have been vaccinated.**"

Dr. Harvey Risch
Professor Epidemiology, Yale University

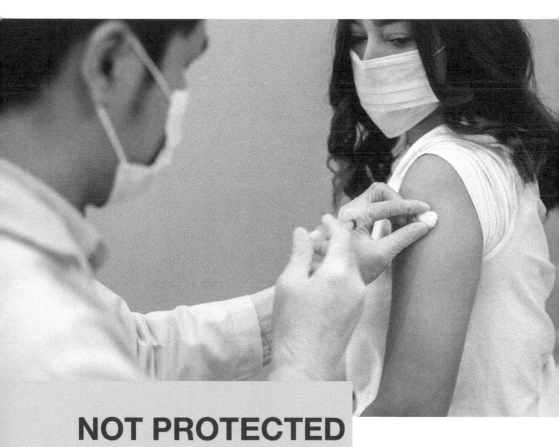

NOT PROTECTED

Breakthrough Infections

As of April 26, the CDC reported

9,245

people had tested positive for COVID at least two weeks after getting their final COVID vaccination.

Why do you think they changed?

CDC is no longer reporting weekly COVID breakthrough infections unless they result in **hospitalization or death.**

CHOOSING YOUR COVID-19 VACCINE
FACTS YOU NEED TO KNOW

Pfizer	**Pfizer:** $4.7 billion in fines for false claims, drug and medical equipment safety violations, off-label promotion, corrupt practices, kickbacks, and bribery.
moderna	**Moderna:** Has never brought a vaccine to market since its founding, despite fielding 9+ vaccine candidates, none of which made it through phase 3 clinical trials.
J&J Johnson&Johnson	**Johnson & Johnson:** Named in hundreds of thousands of lawsuits for toxic and/or dangerous products, including drugs, shampoos, medical equipment, and asbestos-contaminated baby powder.
AstraZeneca	**AstraZeneca:** Suspended by two dozen European countries due to severe, lethal adverse reactions, like blood clots.

Don't worry, you're in safe hands!

If you're vaccinated, remember to wear a mask and socially distance because you can still spread COVID-19. Trust The Science™

READ the HEADLINE below carefully.

Australian Government website

Home > WA Government > Publications >
Public Health Act 2016 (WA) – Instrument of Authorisation – Authorisation to Supply or Administer a Poison [SARS-COV-2 (COVID-19) VACCINE – Australian Defence Force] (No.2) 2021

Public Health Act 2016 (WA) – Instrument of Authorisation – Authorisation to Supply or Administer a Poison [SARS-COV-2 (COVID-19) VACCINE – Australian Defence Force] (No.2) 2021

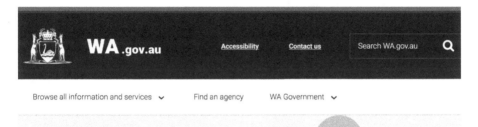

Guidance: An authorisation by the Chief Health Office under the s. 197 and s.198 Public Health Act 2016 (WA) to authorise relevant Australian Defence Force employees to supply and administer the COVID-19 Vaccine.

How these shots can injure you for life.

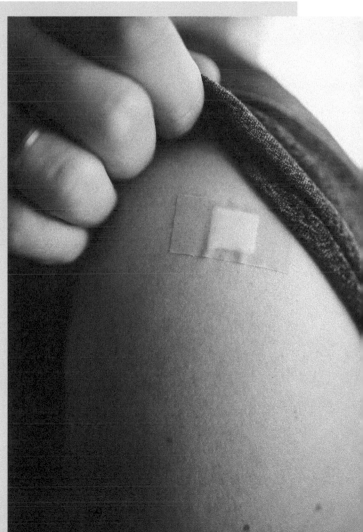

By Dr. Sherri Tenpenny
Cleveland, Ohio

20 Mechanisms of Injuries (MOI)

How COVID-19 Injections Can Make You Sick...Even Kill You

Sherri J. Tenpenny
DO, AOBEM(95-06), AOBNMM, ABIHM

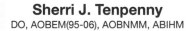

https://www.drtenpenny.com/

28

Tissues Affected

(out of 55 tested)

- Brain
- Immune system
- Pancreas
- Reproductive system
- Testicular tissue
- Placenta
- Ovaries
- Gut and barrier proteins
- Gastrointestinal cells
- Thyroid
- Nervous system
- Heart
- Joint
- Skin
- Muscle
- Mitochondria
- Liver

Study: https://www.ncbi.nlm.nih.gov/pmc/articles/PMC7873987/

https://rumble.com/vepiqt-dr-sherri-tenpenny-and-reinette-senum-march-2021-important-update.html

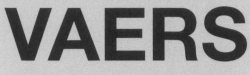

VAERS

Descriptions of Adverse Events

- Anaphylaxis
- Miscarriages
- Paralysis
- Guillain Barre Syndrome
- Sudden Hearing Loss
- Sudden Blindness
- Seizures
- Strokes
- Encephalitis
- Death

https://vaers.hhs.gov/index.html
https://childrenshealthdefense.org/defender/facebook-posts-vaers-link-covid-vaccines-injuries-death/

VAERS
Vaccine Adverse Event Reporting System

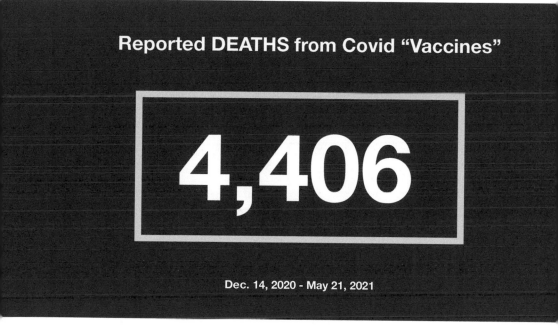

Reported DEATHS from Covid "Vaccines"

4,406

Dec. 14, 2020 - May 21, 2021

● Only ~1% of vaccine reactions reported to **VAERS**

● Reports 2-3 months behind

Lazarus Report: https://digital.ahrq.gov/sites/default/files/docs/publication/
r18hs017045-lazarus-final-report-2011.pdf

https://www.medalerts.org/vaersdb/findfield.php?
TABLE=ON&GROUP1=AGE&EVENTS=ON&VAX=COVID19&DIED=Yes

"Never has a vaccine injured so many"

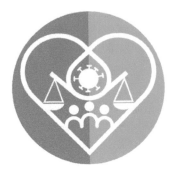

The Israeli People's Committee Report of Adverse Events Related to the Corona Vaccine

April 2021

https://4a1b9d73-4c47-4f3b-bb08-e515be8958ca.filesusr.com/ugd/3db409_3c4b29f97a7b4e2fb1d8d178ab138b91.pdf
https://doctors4covidethics.medium.com/the-israeli-peoples-committee-report-of-adverse-events-related-to-the-corona-vaccine-april-2021-47891f17d452

India's Public Health Ambassador Dies Day After Taking COVID Vaccine

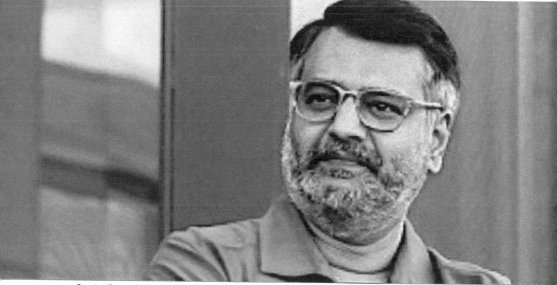

Credit: Great Game India via Twitter

"I want to put an end to all the rumors. I want to show people that there is no danger in getting vaccinated. On the contrary, it will protect us," said Vivekh day before passing.

VAERS
Vaccine Adverse Event Reporting System

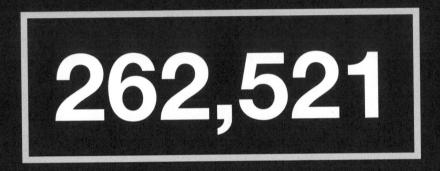

Adverse Events Reported

262,521

Dec. 14, 2020 - May 21, 2021

- Only ~1% of vaccine reactions reported to VAERS

- Reports 2-3 months behind

Lazarus Report: https://digital.ahrq.gov/sites/default/files/docs/publication/r18hs017045-lazarus-final-report-2011.pdf

https://www.medalerts.org/vaersdb/findfield.php?TABLE=ON&GROUP1=CAT&EVENTS=ON&VAX=COVID19

Heart Issues in Teens after Shots

"This was like the first time I thought I was going to die."
16-year old Luke Celic

"He basically has a heart condition now and it's terrifying."
Rachel Hatton, mother of Gregory, 17 years old

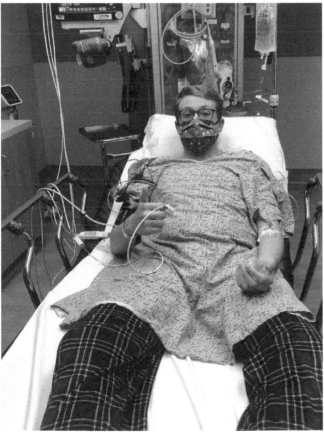

18 hospitalizations in Connecticut

All within 4 days of a Covid shot.

https://www.wfsb.com/news/at-least-18-teens-young-adults-in-ct-experience-heart-issues-after-covid-shot/article_6a34dd80-bcc7-11eb-9c9a-cb35ce5f9763.html

Photo: Twitter, Evan Morud, 18, from Kenmore, WA

the Defender™

CHILDREN'S HEALTH DEFENSE NEWS & VIEWS

05/28/21 • BIG PHARMA › NEWS

COVID Vaccine Injury Reports Among 12- to 17-Year-Olds More Than Triple in 1 Week, VAERS Data Show

VAERS data released today showed 262,521 reports of adverse events following COVID vaccines, including 4,406 deaths and 21,537 serious injuries between Dec. 14, 2020 and May 21, 2021.

HOW TO FILE A REPORT FOR AN ADVERSE EVENT

● **File with VAERS - Governmentt website**
https://vaers.hhs.gov/reportevent.html

● **File with VaxxTracker.com - Independent website**
https://vaxxtracker.com/

● **Report on CHD website (can be anonymous)**
https://childrenshealthdefense.org/covid-19-vaccine-reactions/

https://childrenshealthdefense.org/defender/injured-by-vaccine-how-to-report-it/

https://childrenshealthdefense.org/defender/vaers-data-reports-injuries-12-to-17-year-olds-more-than-triple/?itm_term=home

Reported Deaths Post-COVID Vaccine Total: 4,406

Through May 21, 2021

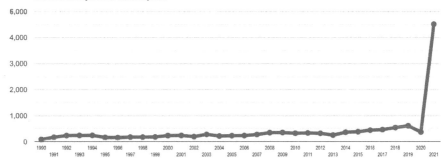

ALL Deaths Reported to VAERS by Year

Source: OpenVaers.com
https://www.openvaers.com/covid-data/mortality

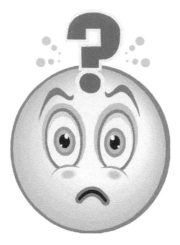

"People think that the side effects of vaccines are harmful, and they get worried when they look at it and read into it, but it's actually a good thing.

It tells us that your immune system is working, and it's responding in the way that we want it to."

- Quote from a Medical Doctor to the Press

"They don't want to see people like us."

Covid Vaccine-Injured Medical Professionals

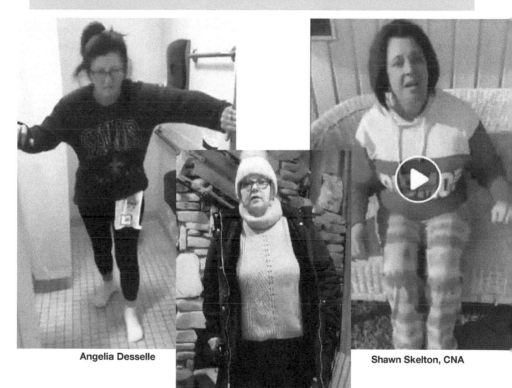

Angelia Desselle

Shawn Skelton, CNA

Kristi Simmonds, RN, NP

MAMMOGRAMS

Screening Facility Message

If you have gotten the COVID-19 Vaccine please call and reschedule 4-6 weeks AFTER the second shot as it will show up in your screening reading.

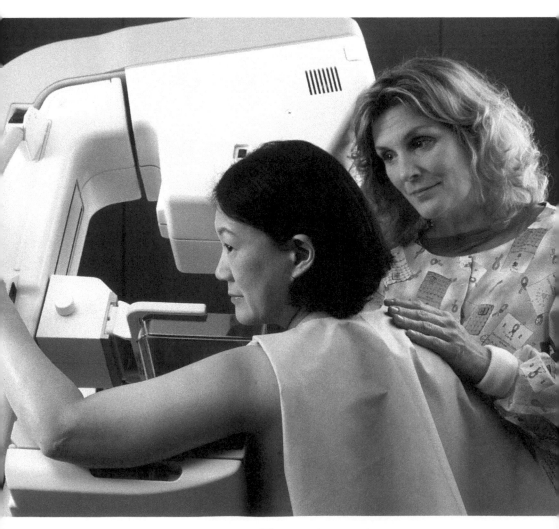

Enlarged lymph nodes LOOK LIKE CANCER and set off a chain of testing.

Long-term effects UNKNOWN

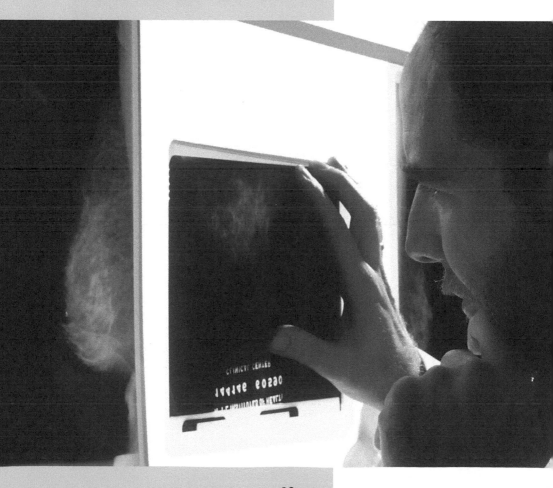

IT'S MAGNETIC!!!

Is this why?

New Discovery:
"Genetically engineered 'Magneto' protein remotely controls brain and behaviour."

https://www.theguardian.com/science/neurophilosophy/2016/mar/24/magneto-remotely-controls-brain-and-behaviour

https://ugetube.com/watch/magnet-challenge-tested-on-random-people-laguna-beach-california-highwire-covid-19-coronavirus-masks_Kh5vac6fo7FzZN1.html

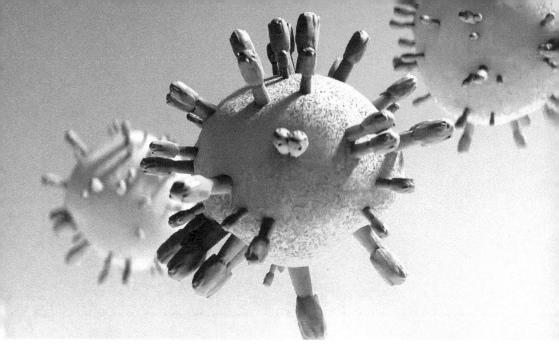

Syncytin arose from a VIRUS.

"So what originally started as a viral gene designed to produce proteins that would fuse the host's cells together, thereby allowing the virus to spread with greater ease, now serves to connect mother and child."

"Quite simply, syncytin is critical and without it, human life could never form."

- Reza Rezaei Javan - I, Science

Syncytin

"There is a striking similarity between human syncytins and the SARS-CoV-2 spike protein.

If the shots create anti-syncytin antibodies, this would prevent the formation of a placenta which would result in *vaccinated* **women essentially becoming**

infertile**"**

**Dr. Michael Yeadon
Dr. Wolfgang Wodarg**

https://cienciaysaludnatural.com/
estudio/why-covid-19-vaccines-might-
affect-fertility/

https://dryburgh.com/wp-content/
uploads/2020/12/
Wodarg_Yeadon_EMA_Petition_Pfiz
er_Trial_FINAL_01DEC2020_signed_
with_Exhibits_geschwarzt.pdf

FOIA Reveals
FOIA - Freedom of Information Act

According to the documents, pre-clinical studies show that the active part of the vaccine (mRNA-lipid nanoparticles), which produce the spike protein, **spreads throughout the body and is then concentrated in various organs, including the ovaries and spleen.** (See chart on the next page)

 The shot approved was a *different* formulation?

Dr. Robert W. Malone, MD, MS
Dr. Malone was the original inventor of the mRNA vaccine technology back in the late 1980s.

Dr. Malone noted that **normal pharmacokinetic and pharmaco-toxicology studies had not been performed before EUA authorization** for the product.

"I was particularly surprised that the dossier of regulatory documents indicates allowance for use in humans based on non-GLP PK and Tox studies relying on **formulations which are significantly different from the final vaccine.**"

https://trialsitenews.com/did-pfizer-fail-to-perform-industry-standard-animal-testing-prior-to-initiation-of-mrna-clinical-trials/

Data on Organ Distribution

2.6.5.5B. PHARMACOKINETICS: ORGAN
DISTRIBUTION CONTINUED

Sample	Total Lipid concentration (µg lipid equivalent/g [or mL]) (males and females combined)						
	0.25 h	1 h	2 h	4 h	8 h	24 h	48 h
Lymph (mandibular)	0.064	0.189	0.290	0.408	0.534	0.554	0.727
Lymph node (mesenteric)	0.050	0.146	0.530	0.489	0.689	0.985	1.37
Muscle	0.021	0.061	0.084	0.103	0.096	0.095	0.192
Ovaries (females)	0.104	1.34	1.64	2.34	3.09	5.24	12.3
Pancreas	0.081	0.207	0.414	0.380	0.294	0.358	0.599
Pituitary gland	0.339	0.645	0.868	0.854	0.405	0.478	0.694
Prostate (males)	0.061	0.091	0.128	0.157	0.150	0.183	0.170
Salivary glands	0.084	0.193	0.255	0.220	0.135	0.170	0.264
Skin	0.013	0.208	0.159	0.145	0.119	0.157	0.253
Small intestine	0.030	0.221	0.476	0.879	1.28	1.30	1.47
Spinal cord	0.043	0.097	0.169	0.250	0.106	0.085	0.112
Spleen	0.334	2.47	7.73	10.3	22.1	20.1	23.4
Stomach	0.017	0.065	0.115	0.144	0.268	0.152	0.215
Tests (Males)	0.031	0.042	0.079	0.129	0.146	0.304	0.320
Thymus	0.088	0.243	0.340	0.335	0.196	0.207	0.331
Thyroid	0.155	0.536	0.842	0.851	0.544	0.578	1.00
Uterus (females)	0.043	0.203	0.305	0.140	0.287	0.289	0.456
Whole blood	1.97	4.37	5.40	3.05	1.31	0.909	0.420
Plasma	3.97	8.13	8.90	6.50	2.36	1.78	0.805
Blood: plasma ratio	0.815	0.515	0.550	0.510	0.555	0.530	0.540

The Spike Protein can attach to the ACE2 Receptor on the surface of the sperm.

● **WHAT IF** the spike protein is in the vagina?

● **WHAT IF** THAT particular sperm fertilizes the egg?

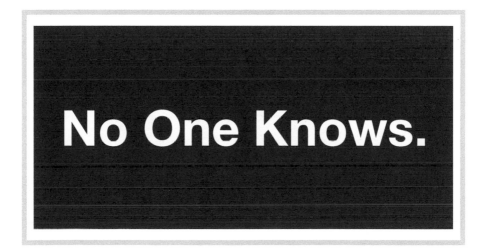

No One Knows.

Sherri J. Tenpenny
DO, AOBEM(95-06), AOBNMM, ABIHM

https://www.drtenpenny.com/

Number of reported Miscarriages to MHRA due to AstraZeneca Vaccine increases by 550% in just eight weeks

BY THE DAILY EXPOSE ON APRIL 2, 2021 • (1 COMMENT)

+550%

UK

December 9, 2020 - March 21, 2021

https://dailyexpose.co.uk/2021/04/02/number-of-reported-miscarriages-to-mhra-due-to-astrazeneca-vaccine-increases-by-550-in-just-eight-weeks/

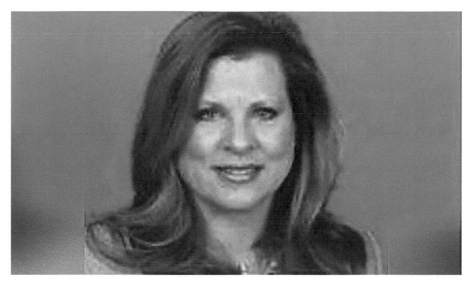

Dr. Janci Chunn Lindsay
in a public comment to the CDC on 4/23/21

"We could potentially sterilize an entire generation."

These injections "must be halted immediately."

Thousands of Reports

Decidual Casts

You can even see the
ridges of the uterus.

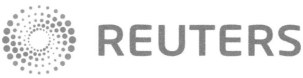

REUTERS

Brazil suspends use of AstraZeneca vaccine in pregnant women nationally after death

BRASILIA/RIO DE JANEIRO (Reuters) -Brazil's federal government on Tuesday nationally suspended the vaccination of pregnant women with the AstraZeneca COVID-19 shot, after an expectant mother in Rio de Janeiro died from a stroke possibly related to the inoculation.

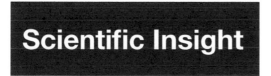

Scientific Insight

"When RNA contains more cytosine (C) and more guanine (G), it's more likely to be able to make protein. So the V's mRNA was manipulated to have lots of C's and G's so it could produce 1,000 times as much spike protein.

The resulting spike protein that is produced was made to fold differently than if you had gotten the natural virus. The spike protein that is produced by your body after getting the V is made with proline which is a very stiff amino acid that doesn't move. It sticks to the ACE-2 receptor, it doesn't go anywhere.

That's going to suppress ACE-2 and that's how you get pulmonary hypertension, you get ventricular heart failure, you get stroke."
                                    - Dr. Stephanie Seneff, MIT

https://news.yahoo.com/brazil-health-agency-calls-halt-110722688.html

Facebook Fertility Clinic Posts

- Incredible amount of miscarriages.

- All male sperm from vx people is sterile

- All embryos failed to fertilize

"It is unprecedented."

Lethal event for the fetus.

● **18 weeks pregnant**
Pfizer Vaccine 1/12/21
Baby Stillborn 6 days later

This is VAERS ID 958755

Case Details

VAERS ID: 958755 (history) **Vaccinated:** 2021-01-12
Form: Version 2.0 **Onset:** 2021-01-18
Age: 40.0 **Days after vaccination:** 6
Sex: Female **Submitted:** 0000-00-00
Location: California **Entered:** 2021-01-20

Vaccination / Manufacturer	Lot / Dose	Site / Route
COVID19: COVID19 (COVID19 (PFIZER-BIONTECH)) / PFIZER/BIONTECH	EK9231 4/21 / 1	- / IM

Administered by: Unknown **Purchased by:** ?
Symptoms: Exposure during pregnancy, Foetal death, Premature delivery, Premature separation of placenta, Stillbirth, Ultrasound antenatal screen normal, Vaginal haemorrhage
SMQs:, Haemorrhage terms (excl laboratory terms) (narrow), Pregnancy, labour and delivery complications and risk factors (excl abortions and stillbirth) (narrow), Termination of pregnancy and risk of abortion (narrow), Normal pregnancy conditions and outcomes (narrow)
Life Threatening? Yes
Birth Defect? No
Died? No
Permanent Disability? No
Recovered? Yes
Office Visit? No
ER Visit? No
ER or Doctor Visit? No
Hospitalized? Yes, 1 days
   Extended hospital stay? No
Previous Vaccinations:
Other Medications: prenatal vitamins
Current Illness: none
Preexisting Conditions: none
Allergies: none
Diagnostic Lab Data:
CDC Split Type:
Write-up: Pt was 18 weeks pregnant at the time of the vaccine. Second pregnancy. Pt is a physician. Pregnancy was entirely normal up to that time. On 1/18/2021, she began to have heavy vaginal bleeding probably due to a placental abruption and subsequently delivered at 18 weeks. Baby was stillborn. Ultrasound done 1/15/2021 normal. Lethal event for the fetus. The patient did well.

https://www.lifesitenews.com/news/thousands-of-women-report-hemorrhaging-reproductive-dysfunction-miscarriage-after-corona-shots

3 YEAR-OLD

Bleeding and Passing Clots

😈damn it Ladies....another urgent appt for 6 tonight just called because 3 yr old girl around her vaxxed grandmother this weekend. Parents need to bring her in asap because she's bleeding, passing clots, in pain & getting lesions around her lips.

I can't tell ya'll how many times I've needed to vomit during appts these past 2 weeks.

Doctors for Covid Ethics

Over 100 Doctors and Scientists from 25 countries

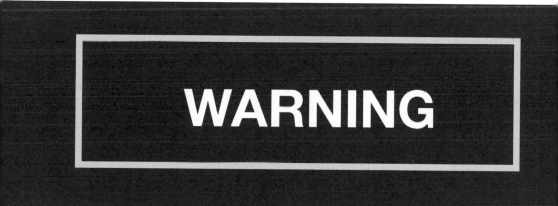

Clotting and bleeding after vaccination can also **"be expected to increase with each re-vaccination, and each intervening coronavirus exposure."**

https://doctors4covidethics.medium.com/rebuttal-letter-to-european-medicines-agency-from-doctors-for-covid-ethics-april-1-2021-7d867f0121e

My Cycle Story

An Independent Research Study Collecting Data Around Women's Cycle Changes

We want to make sure that women are being heard. We are a group of concerned data analysts, doctors, lawyers, scientists and citizens who are coming together in agreement that there is "something" happening and there is no one doing a thorough investigation on this issue.

Participating in this study will involve completing a secure online survey which takes about 15-20 minutes.

Help Us Find the Answers with Your Cycle Story

mycyclestory.com

Visit the Question section of our site for information about how we are ensuring your privacy is protected.

- **Abnormal Periods**

- **Heavy Bleeding**

- **Miscarriages**

- **Sperm Not Motile**

What's Going On?

Self-Spreading Vaccines

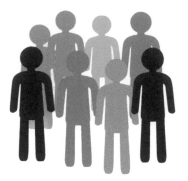

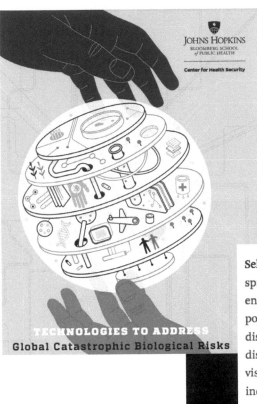

Self-Spreading Vaccines: Self-spreading vaccines are genetically engineered to move through populations like communicable diseases, but rather than causing disease, they confer protection. The vision is that a small number of individuals in a target population could be vaccinated, and the vaccine strain would then circulate in the population much like a pathogenic virus, resulting in rapid, widespread immunity.

See the John Hopkins Report Here

https://jhsphcenterforhealthsecurity.s3.amazonaws.com/
181009-gcbr-tech-report.pdf

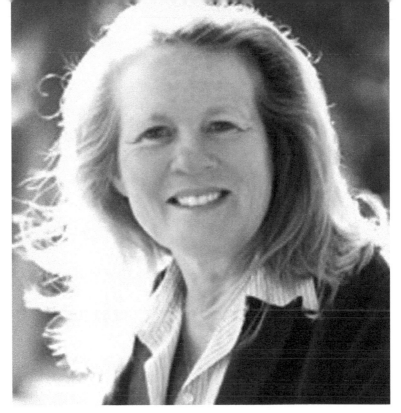

Judy Mikovits, Ph.D.
Cellular and Molecular Biologist

Self-Spreading Vaccines

"Micro RNA's can be **inhaled or driven through the skin** and **change the regulation of the endocrine system.**

Lipid nanoparticles in Gardasil are similar."

https://ijvtpr.com/index.php/IJVTPR/article/view/23

https://soundcloud.com/robin-westenra/judy-mikovits-spike-protein-shedding-crisis-the-panic-is-spreading

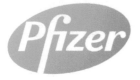

Pfizer Clinical Protocol C4591001

10.4. Appendix 4: Contraceptive Guidance 10.4.1.

Male Participant Reproductive Inclusion Criteria Male participants are eligible to participate if they agree to the following requirements during the intervention period and for at least

28 days after the last dose of study intervention, which corresponds to the time needed to eliminate reproductive safety risk of the study intervention(s):

- Must agree to use a male condom when engaging in any activity that allows for passage of ejaculate to another person.

- In addition to male condom use, a highly effective method of contraception may be considered in WOCBP partners of male participants

  (refer to the list of highly effective methods below in Section 10.4.4).

What is WOCBP?
Women Of Childbearing Potential

See the Pfizer Clinical Protocol Here

https://web.archive.org/web/20200928044805/https://pfe-pfizercom-d8-prod.s3.amazonaws.com/2020-09/C4591001_Clinical_Protocol.pdf

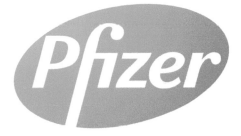

Pfizer Clinical Protocol C4591001
8.3.5.1. Exposure During Pregnancy

A female is found to be pregnant while being exposed or having been exposed to study intervention due to environmental exposure. Below are examples of environmental exposure during pregnancy:

Exposure Concern

• A female family member or healthcare provider reports that she is pregnant after having been exposed to the study intervention by **inhalation or skin contact.**

Exposure Concern

• A male family member or healthcare provider who has been exposed to the study intervention by inhalation or skin contact then exposes his female partner prior to or around the time of conception. or healthcare provider who has been exposed to the study intervention by **inhalation or skin contact** then exposes his female partner prior to or around the time of conception.

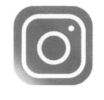

VA((INATED

One of the creative spellings of VACCINATED
used to avoid censorship.

OVER TWENTY THOUSAND
WOMEN WERE IN A GROUP
REPORTING REPRODUCTIVE
ISSUES AFTER BEING EXPOSED
TO A VA((INATED PERSON AND
THE GROUP WAS DELETED BY
FACEBOOK YESTERDAY.

LET THAT SINK IN.

Patent: Fertility Impairing Vaccine and Method Of Use

Developed for dogs and cats.

PCT

WORLD INTELLECTUAL PROPERTY ORGANIZATION
International Bureau

INTERNATIONAL APPLICATION PUBLISHED UNDER THE PATENT COOPERATION TREATY (PCT)

(51) International Patent Classification [6]: A61K 39/00, 39/39	**A1**	**(11) International Publication Number:** WO 99/34825
		(43) International Publication Date: 15 July 1999 (15.07.99)

(21) International Application Number: PCT/US98/27658

(22) International Filing Date: 30 December 1998 (30.12.98)

(30) Priority Data:
60/070,375	2 January 1998 (02.01.98)	US
60/071,406	15 January 1998 (15.01.98)	US
60/076,368	27 February 1998 (27.02.98)	US

(71) Applicant *(for all designated States except US):* THE UNIVERSITY OF GEORGIA RESEARCH FOUNDATION, INC. [US/US]; Boyd Graduate Studies Research Center, Athens, GA 30602-7411 (US).

(72) Inventor; and
(75) Inventor/Applicant *(for US only):* FAYRER–HOSKEN, Richard, A. [US/US]; P.O. Box 27, Winterville, GA 30683 (US).

(74) Agent: SANDBERG, Victoria, A.; Mueting, Raasch & Gebhardt, P.O. Box 581415, Minneapolis, MN 55458–1415 (US).

(81) Designated States: AL, AM, AT, AU, AZ, BA, BB, BG, BR, BY, CA, CH, CN, CU, CZ, DE, DK, EE, ES, FI, GB, GD, GE, GH, HU, IL, IS, JP, KE, KG, KP, KR, KZ, LC, LK, LR, LS, LT, LU, LV, MD, MG, MK, MN, MW, MX, NO, NZ, PL, PT, RO, RU, SD, SE, SG, SI, SK, SL, TJ, TM, TR, TT, UA, UG, US, UZ, VN, YU, ZW, ARIPO patent (GH, GM, KE, LS, MW, SD, SZ, UG, ZW), Eurasian patent (AM, AZ, BY, KG, KZ, MD, RU, TJ, TM), European patent (AT, BE, CH, CY, DE, DK, ES, FI, FR, GB, GR, IE, IT, LU, MC, NL, PT, SE), OAPI patent (BF, BJ, CF, CG, CI, CM, GA, GN, GW, ML, MR, NE, SN, TD, TG).

Published
With international search report.
With amended claims.

ITY IMPAIRING VACCINE AND METHOD OF USE

And ... Humans!

"The observed ovarian dysfunction, often associated with immunization by ZP glycoproteins, is one of the major obstacles for their application in

the control of human population."

SOURCE for the Study

"Update on zona pellucida glycoproteins based contraceptive vaccine."

https://pubmed.ncbi.nlm.nih.gov/15288184/

Project Coast:

Apartheid's Chemical and Biological Warfare Programme

Chandré Gould and Peter Folb

Edited by Robert Berold

UNIDIR
United Nations Institute for Disarmament Research
Geneva, Switzerland

CCR
Centre for Conflict Resolution
Cape Town, South Africa

https://www.unidir.org/files/publications/pdfs/project-coast-apartheid-s-chemical-and-biological-warfare-programme-296.pdf

From the Project Coast Report

"Dr Daniel Goosen. Goosen, who had done research into embryo transplants, told the TRC that he and Basson had discussed the possibility of developing an anti-fertility vaccine which could be selectively administered — **without the knowledge of the recipient.** The intention, he said, was to administer it to black South African women without their knowledge. This was confirmed by Dr Schalk Van Rensburg who oversaw the fertility project."

"The researchers thought that if the formation of HCG in women shortly after conception could be prevented, **the result would be effective contraception.**"

https://www.unidir.org/files/publications/pdfs/project-coast-apartheid-s-chemical-and-biological-warfare-programme-296.pdf

Mass Sterilization
Kenyan Doctors Find Anti-Fertility Agent In UN Tetanus Vaccine

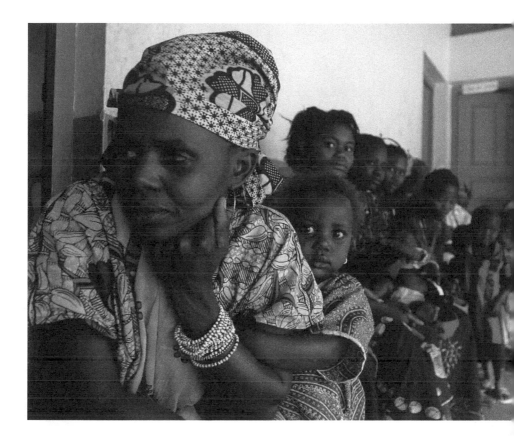

AFRICAN GLOBE – According to a report, the Kenya Catholic Doctors Association is charging UNICEF and WHO with **sterilizing millions of girls and women under cover of an anti-tetanus vaccination program sponsored by the Kenyan government.**

Samples tested positive for the **HCG antigen.**

2014-2015

Credits: Pierre Holtz for UNICEF | www.hdptcar.net

https://www.kenya-today.com/news/catholic-warning-neonatal-tetanus-vaccine-wto-deadly-bad-women-reproductivity

What Else Could Possibly Go WRONG?

Can the shots permanently alter DNA?

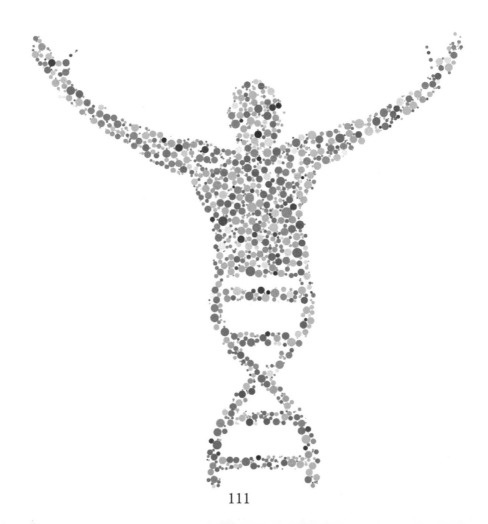

Prelim Studies Suggest DNA Is Altered

 "SARS-CoV-2 RNA reverse-transcribed and integrated into the human genome."

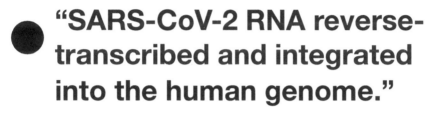 Harvard–MIT
Health Sciences & Technology

 "Modified RNA has a direct effect on DNA stability."

 UiO :

University of Oslo

https://phys.org/news/2020-01-rna-effect-dna.html
https://www.biorxiv.org/content/biorxiv/early/2020/12/13/2020.12.12.422516.full.pdf

PRION DISEASE

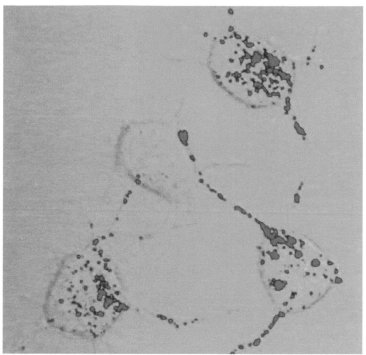

Prion protein (stained in red) revealed in a photomicrograph of neural tissue from a scrapie-infected mouse.

"We identified the presence of prion-like domains in the SARS-CoV-2 spike protein."

Prions: **unprecedented infectious pathogens** that cause a group of fatal neurodegenerative diseases by a novel mechanism. They are **transmissible particles** that are devoid of nucleic acid.

In Humans: Creutzfeldt-Jakob diseases
In Bovines: Mad Cow Disease

https://www.preprints.org/manuscript/202003.0422/v1
https://principia-scientific.com/covid-19-rna-based-vaccines-and-the-risk-of-prion-disease/
https://carterheavyindustries.files.wordpress.com/2021/02/covid19-rna-based-vaccines-and-the-risk-of-prion-disease-1503.pdf

Predictive Programming?

 Centers for Disease Control and Prevention
CDC 24/7: Saving Lives, Protecting People™

Search

A-Z

Advanced S

Center for Preparedness and Response

Center for Preparedness and Response

🔘 About Us

🏠 Center for Preparedness
and Response

About Us

What We Do   +

Why it Matters

Who We Are   +

Emergency Preparedness
Funding

Prepare Your Health

Emergency Operations   +

Zombie Preparedness

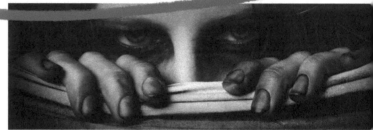

Wonder why zombies, zombie apocalypse, and zombie preparedness continue to live or walk dea
a CDC web site? As it turns out what first began as a tongue-in-cheek campaign to engage new
audiences with preparedness messages has proven to be a very effective platform. We continue t
reach and engage a wide variety of audiences on all hazards preparedness via "zombie

- **Zombie Preparedness Blog**
- **Zombie Preparedness for Educators**
- **Zombie Preparedness Poster**
- **Zombie Preparedness Graphic Novel**

Don't Believe It?
Check it out: CDC Official Website
https://www.cdc.gov/cpr/zombie/index.htm

Third COVID Wave Will Kill Or Hospitalize 60 to 70% Of People Who Took Both The Vaccine Doses Says Official UK Govt Model

Figure 11: Results of the central scenario of the Warwick model, showing the age and vaccine status of those admitted to hospital (left) or dying (right) over time. Top plots are absolute numbers, bottom plots are proportions.

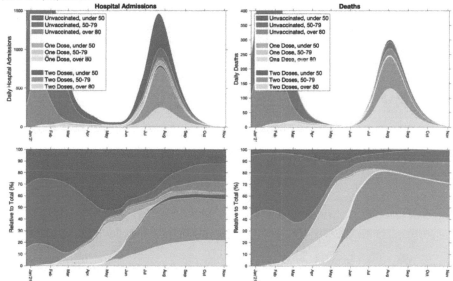

UK Government Recommendation
Lockdowns Until Variant Vaccine Available

ADE

**Antibody-Dependent Enhancement
Pathogenic Priming**

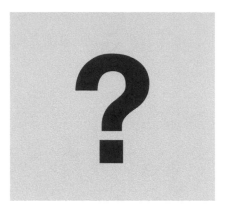

Why have coronavirus vaccines *never* been approved for humans in the last 20 years?

Laboratory animals tested contracted more serious symptoms upon re-infection and most of them DIED.

 WILL THIS BE THE THIRD WAVE?

https://pubmed.ncbi.nlm.nih.gov/22536382/

https://www.frontiersin.org/articles/10.3389/fimmu.2021.640093/full#B77

https://dryburgh.com/wp-content/uploads/2020/12/
Wodarg_Yeadon_EMA_Petition_Pfizer_Trial_FINAL_01DEC2020_signed_with_Exhibits_geschwarzt.pdf

https://coronanews123.wordpress.com/2021/01/25/the-coming-genocide-of-adverse-covid-vax-reactions-and-who-to-blame-for-it/

FAQ's

Are the vaccines experimental? YES

Will the vaccines stop me from getting COVID? NO

Will the vaccines stop me from spreading COVID? NO

Have the vaccines caused any deaths or injuries? YES

Are the vaccine manufacturers liable for injuries or deaths caused by the vaccines? NO

Covid 19 Survival Rates
CDC - September 10, 2020

Age	Survival Rate
0-19	**99.997%**
20-49	**99.98%**
50-69	**99.5%**
70 +	**94.6%**
Flu All Ages	**99.89%**

https://projectwaistline.com/?p=21863
https://lbry.tv/@SixthSense-Truth-Search-Labs:0/covid-survival-rates-poster:4
https://www.cdc.gov/coronavirus/2019-ncov/hcp/planning-scenarios.html

Swine Flu

October 1976 - December 1976

40 Million Americans Vaccinated

500 Cases of Paralysis

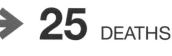 **25** DEATHS

Program stopped Dec. 16, 1976

COVID

December 14, 2020 -May 13, 2021

119 Million Americans Fully Vaccinated

262,521 VAERS (Dec. 14 - May 21, 2021)

4,406 DEATHS

First **1,600 Deaths** have been evaluated by the CDC and said to be **unrelated to the vaccine.**

https://www.cdc.gov/coronavirus/2019-ncov/covid-data/covidview/index.html
https://www.ncbi.nlm.nih.gov/pmc/articles/PMC1436986/pdf/jrsocmed00281-0040.pdf
https://sciencebasedmedicine.org/the-covid-19-vaccine-holocaust-the-latest-antivaccine-messaging/

57 Top Scientists and Doctors: Stop All Covid Vaccinations

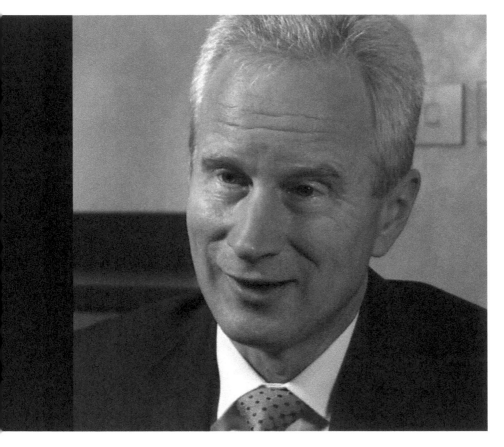

Peter A. McCullough, MD, MPH
Internist, Cardiologist, Epidemiologist & Professor of Medicine

SARS-CoV-2 mass vaccination: **Urgent questions on vaccine safety that demand answers from international health agencies, regulatory authorities, governments and vaccine developers.**

COVID is a Crime Against Humanity

1,000 Lawyers and 10,000 Doctors led by Dr. Reiner Fuellmich have begun legal proceedings against the CDC, WHO and the Davos Group for crimes against humanity.

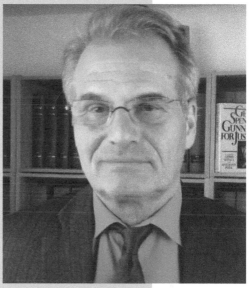

Dr. Reiner Fuellmich

⚫ They present the faulty PCR test and the order for doctors to label any comorbidity death as a Covid death as fraud.

⚫ The "experimental" vaccine is in violation of all 10 of the Nuremberg Codes which carry the death penalty for those who seek to violate these International Laws.

https://alethonews.com/2021/05/07/covid-fraud-legal-proceedings-begin-against-w-h-o-and-world-leaders-for-crimes-against-humanity/

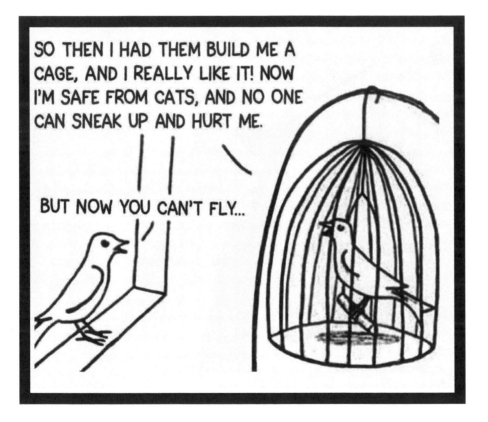

Join The Health Freedom Movement

Millions Against Medical Mandates
mamm.org

National Vaccine Information Center (NVIC)
nvic.org

Children's Health Defense (CHD)
childrenshealthdefense.org

Mercola.com

Informed Consent Action Network (ICAN)
icandecide.org

Vaxxter
vaxxter.com

Green Med Info
greenmedinfo.com

America's Frontline Doctors
americasfrontlinedoctors.org

Make Americans Free Again
makeamericansfreeagain.com

Age of Autism
ageofautism.com

Advocates for
Health Freedom

Sherri J. Tenpenny, DO	Vladimir Zelenko, MD
Judy A. Mikovits, PhD	Pierre Kory, MD, MPA
Joseph Mercola, DO	Ryan Cole, MD
Rashid Buttar, DO	Ben Tapper, DC
Dolores Cahill, PhD	Kelly Brogan, MD
Carrie Madej, DO	Thomas Cowan, MD
Jim Meehan, MD	Paul Thomas, MD
Larry Palevsky, MD	Kevin Jenkins, CEO
Lee Merrit, MD	Sucharit Bhakdi, MD
Richard Bartlett, MD	Peter McCullough, MD
Scott Jensen, MD	Sayer Ji, GreenMedInfo

Treatments

This critical information comes from courageous doctors whose integrity is still intact even though they face serious personal threats and are being targeted by groups intent on censoring and disparaging them.

They are heroes.

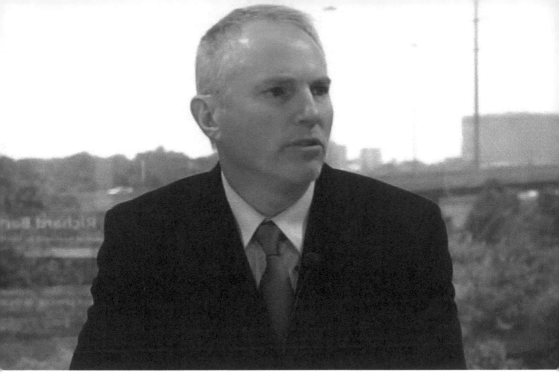

Dr. Richard Bartlett

- **Over 20 years in Family Medicine**
- **Discovered Budesonide as a Covid-19 Treatment**

"Inhaled Budesonide has been studied and utilized for lung-related inflammation for over 20+ years and is safe enough for 2-pound infants in the NICU."

"Thus far, **100% of my patients appear to be symptom-free** following a course of inhaled Budesonide therapy."

https://www.ox.ac.uk/news/2021-02-09-common-asthma-treatment-reduces-need-hospitalisation-covid-19-patients-study

https://www.thethinkingconservative.com/dr-richard-bartlett-on-budesonide-the-silver-bullet-covid-treatment/

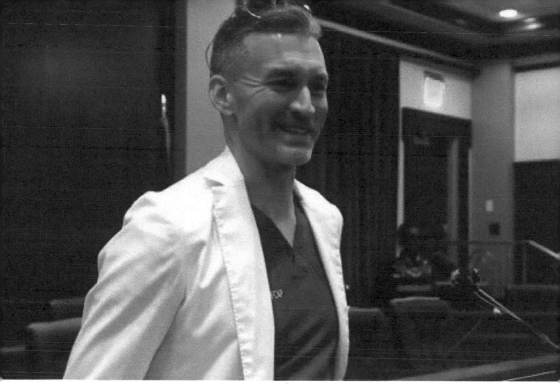

Dr. Ryan Cole

- **Mayo Clinic trained Board Certified Pathologist**
- **CEO and Medical Director of Cole Diagnostics, one of the largest independent labs in Idaho**

The Public Health Message should be about 3 things:

1.Vitamin D
2.Vitamin D
3.Vitamin D

https://www.youtube.com/watch?v=vdrRGmoTYv4

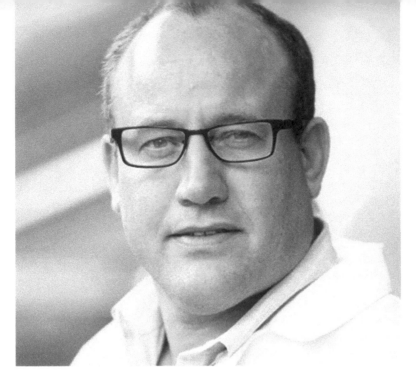

Dr. Pierre Kory

- Board Certified in Critical Medicine, Pulmonary Diseases and Internal Medicine.
- Board Certified Pathologist
- Chief of the Critical Care Service, Medical Director of the Trauma and Life Support Center, University of Wisconsin
- He has worked closely with COVID-19 patients across the US throughout the pandemic.

"The virus can't infect, can't replicate and can't kill you if you're on

Ivermectin.

It absolutely blocks the replication of the SARS-CoV-2 virus."

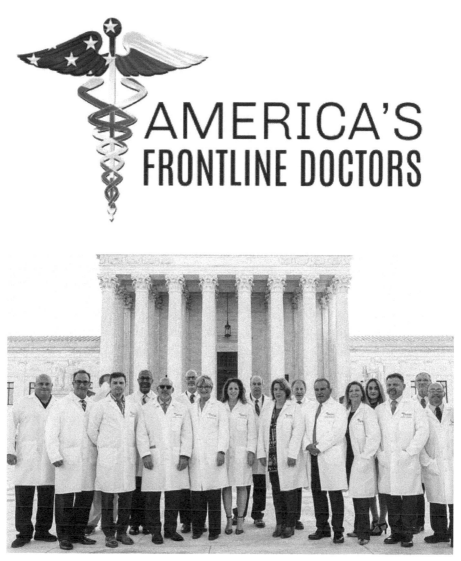

photo: AFLDS.org

Telemedicine Services and Medications

https://www.americasfrontlinedoctors.org/

Information and Protocols

America's Frontline Doctors

AFLDS White Paper: Experimental Vaccines for COVID-19
assets.website-files.com/606d3a50c62e44338008303d/
6076e4fd8bde421370729e47_Vaccine-PP.pdf

AFLDS White Paper on HCQ 2020
americasfrontlinedoctors.com/wp-content/uploads/
2020/09/White-Paper-on-HCQ-2020.2.pdf

FLCCC Alliance - Paul E. Marik, M.D., FCCM, FCCP
Pierre Kory, M.D. M.P.A. | G. Umberto Meduri, M.D.
Joseph Varon, M.D., FCCP, FCCM | Jose Igelsias, D.O.

COVID-19 Protocols
MASK+ Prevention & Early Outpatient Protocol
MATH+ Hospital Treatment Protocol
covid19criticalcare.com/covid-19-protocols

Richard Bartlett, M.D., Budesonide Protocol
aestheticsadvisor.com/2021/04/dr-richard-bartlett-
budesonide-protocol.html

Directory of Doctors Prescribing Effective Outpatient COVID-19 Therapy
exstnc.com

MyFreeDoctor.com
myfreedoctor.com

Rapid Virus Recovery

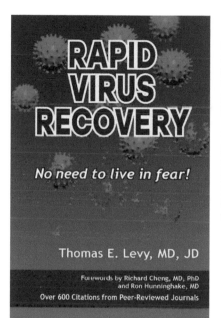

It turns out that there are many remedies that directly use and stimulate the body's natural ability to kill pathogens. Particularly for COVID and other acutely contracted respiratory viruses, the treatments can be incredibly quick as well as effective.

The primary treatment discussed in this book is easy to take and literally costs only pennies. There are no toxic side effects, and it is readily available to anyone. Dr. Levy's new book provides practical instruction on how to instill hydrogen peroxide into the respiratory system via nebulization.

Free Copy Available

rvr.medfoxpub.com

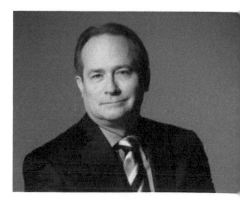

Thomas E. Levy, MD, JD, is a board-certified cardiologist and the author of "Curing the Incurable: Vitamin C, Infectious Diseases, and Toxins" and "STOP America's #1 Killer!" plus several other groundbreaking medical books.

He is one of the world's leading vitamin C experts and frequently lectures to medical professionals all over the globe about the proper role of vitamin C and antioxidants in the treatment of a host of medical conditions and diseases.

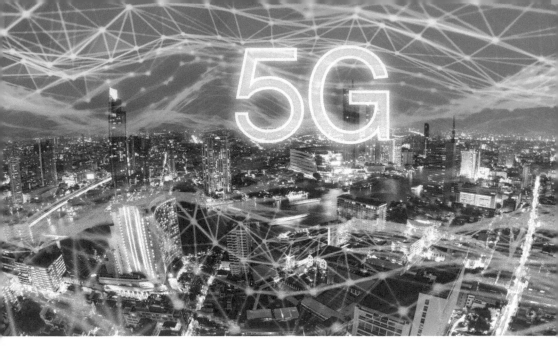

The Environmental Health Trust has termed 5G

"the next great unknown experiment on our children"— and the entire human population.

"... children who began using either cordless or mobile phones regularly before age 20 had more than a **fourfold increased brain tumor risk.**"

WATCH ehtrust.org

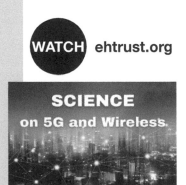

SCIENCE
on 5G and Wireless.

https://childrenshealthdefense.org/news/the-dangers-of-5g-to-childrens-health/

It's All About Controlling Frequency

Patent: Subliminal acoustic manipulation of nervous systems

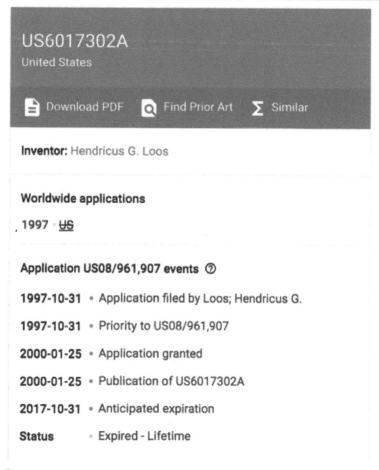

US6017302A
United States

Download PDF   Find Prior Art   Σ Similar

Inventor: Hendricus G. Loos

Worldwide applications

1997 · US

Application US08/961,907 events ⑦

1997-10-31 • Application filed by Loos; Hendricus G.

1997-10-31 • Priority to US08/961,907

2000-01-25 • Application granted

2000-01-25 • Publication of US6017302A

2017-10-31 • Anticipated expiration

Status • Expired - Lifetime

HUMAN ANTENNA - BROADCASTING THE VACCINE FREQUENCY - DAVID ICKE https://www.bitchute.com/video/6r4fMS6aQ9Kn/

VACCINE INFORMATION

Package Inserts
HopkinsVaccine.org
immunize.org/fda

Vaccine Ingredients
https://www.cdc.gov/vaccines/pubs/pinkbook/downloads/
appendices/B/excipient-table-2.pdf

Vaccine Information Statements (VIS)
https://www.cdc.gov/vaccines/hcp/vis/index.html?s_cid=cs_74

Vaccine Injury Table
https://www.hrsa.gov/sites/default/files/vaccinecompensation/
pre03202017-vaccineinjurytable.pdf

Vaccine Adverse Event Reporting System
Government site
https://vaers.hhs.gov/

VaxxTracker.com
Independent site for reporting any side-effect
https://vaxxtracker.com/

Childrens Health Defense
Information and report reactions - can be anonymous
https://childrenshealthdefense.org/covid-19-vaccine-reactions/

Hear This Well: Breaking the Silence on Vaccine Violence
https://www.youtube.com/channel/UCFCrfK5rP_
B6huriP1hLApw/videos

International Memorial for Vaccine Victims
https://www.nvic.org/Vaccine-Memorial.aspx

RESOURCES

20 Mechanisms of Injury Ebook
By Dr. Sherri Tenpenny
drtenpenny.com/product-page/20-mechanisms-of-injury-ebook

Thimerosal, Let the Science Speak: The Evidence Supporting the Immediate Removal of Mercury-a Known Neurotoxin-from Vaccines.
By Robert F. Kennedy Jr.

Expert evaluation on adverse effects of the Pfizer-COVID-19 vaccination
americasfrontlinedoctors.org/frontline-news/expert-evaluation
-on-adverse-effects-of-the-pfizer-covid-19-vaccination

Why Wearing a Mask Makes Healthy People Sick
MeehanMD.com

MMS Health Recovery Guidebook
jimhumblebooks.co/product/mms-health-recovery-guidebook-
2016-paperback

Saliva Tests, Alliance for Natural Health
anhinternational.org/news/covid-tests-in-school-could-
harm-or-mislead

Computational evaluation of major components from plant essential oils as potent inhibitors of SARS-CoV-2 spike protein.
pubmed.ncbi.nlm.nih.gov/32834111

COVID VACCINE MANUFACTURER FACT SHEETS

PFIZER-BIONTECH COVID-19 VACCINE
fda.gov/media/144414/download

COVID-19 Vaccine AstraZeneca
tga.gov.au/sites/default/files/cmi-approved-covid19-vaccine-az.pdf

MODERNA COVID-19 VACCINE
fda.gov/media/144637/download

JANSSEN COVID-19 VACCINE
fda.gov/media/146305/download

THE HUMAN
EMOTIONAL VIBRATION CHART

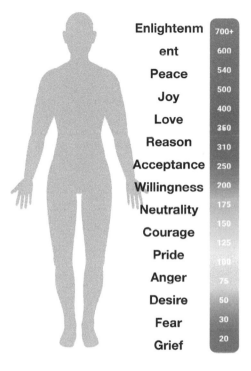

Enlightenment	700+
	600
Peace	540
	500
Joy	
	400
Love	
	350
Reason	310
Acceptance	250
Willingness	200
Neutrality	175
	150
Courage	
	125
Pride	100
Anger	75
Desire	50
Fear	30
Grief	20

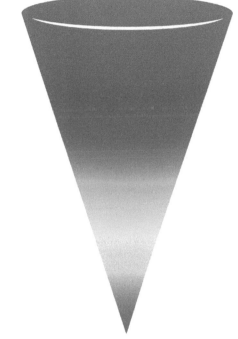

"THE LAST THING STANDING BETWEEN A CHILD AND INDUSTRY CORRUPTION IS A MOM."

-RFK, JR.

Sing, play music, breathe deeply.

Practice intermittent fasting.
Take saunas.
Get out in the sunlight.
Stand barefoot on the ground regularly.
Expand your energy field.

Your power rests in your ability to stay positive and healthy, but also to see the truth behind what is really going on.

Getting stuck in anger, fear, or revenge won't do you or anyone else any good.

You need to enjoy your life now as much as possible and not get bogged down in the conflict that is all around.

Stay neutral. You have no idea what the soul journey of another is meant to be.

You are made of Divine Radiant substance. The very stuff of creation. And you have the ability to command Divine Radiant Substances to manifest for you in glorious ways.

That is the power of each of us as humans connected with the Creator.

- Christiane Northrup, M.D.

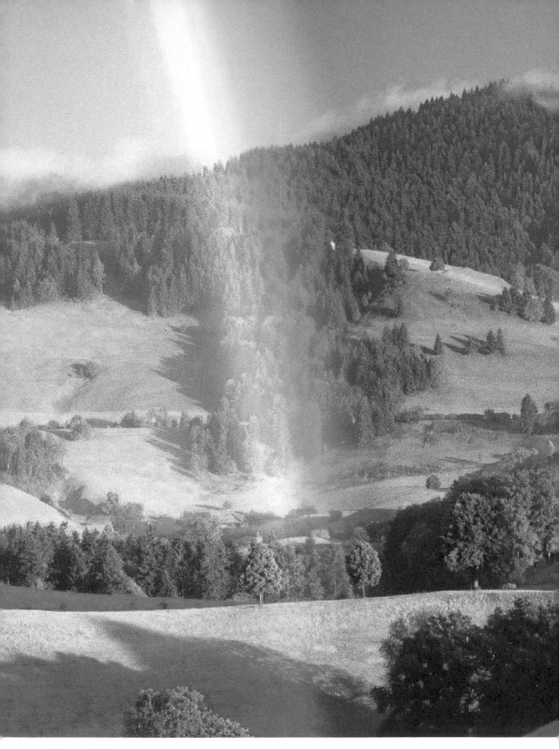

drnorthrup.com

Proceeds from this book will go to www.MaineStandsUp.org, an affiliate of
www.makeamericansfreeagain.com. We stand for health freedom and human rights.

Special thanks to Mary Zakrasek, PhD